# RHEUMATOID ARTHRITIS RELIEF DIET COOKBOOK:

## Revitalize Your Plate, Relieve Your Joints

## Dr. VERA J. REYNOLD

# CONTENTS

# INTRODUCTION

In the symphony of life, the balance between health and pleasure is frequently sought but never attained. Enter the "Rheumatoid Arthritis Diet Cookbook," a grand opus precisely prepared to choreograph a culinary experience that exceeds the borders of feeding and stretches into the realm of healing.

Imagine a world where every meal that graces your table isn't simply a feast for the senses and a balm for your body. In these pages, you'll discover a library of recipes that pay respect to the beauty of cooking while keeping a close eye on the requirements of individuals navigating the complicated roads of rheumatoid arthritis.

At the core of this rich cookbook is the concept that food is not only sustenance; it's medicine. The alchemy turns a plain meal into a rite of rejuvenation. As you explore the tempting alternatives inside, you'll begin a voyage of self-discovery, embracing tastes that connect with your body's well-being.

From dawn's first light to the twilight's warm embrace, every chapter unfolds like a new day of gastronomic adventure. Dive into breakfast delicacies that feed your palette and your joints. Traverse through meals that are an oasis of inflammation-soothing sustenance. Indulge in feasts that highlight both taste and harmony. And when the day winds down, take refuge in sweets that satisfy your taste senses while honouring your body's requirements.

But this cookbook isn't just about recipes; it's a trip of empowerment. Beyond the delectable recipes, you'll uncover insights that elucidate the delicate link between nutrition and rheumatoid arthritis. Discover the function of inflammation-fighting nutrients and how to make balanced, nutrient-packed meals that respond to your body's needs.

Picture this: armed with a spatula, you build a road to health that's as tasty as it is intentional. Here, the kitchen isn't simply a place to cook; it's a sanctuary where every chop, stir, and sizzle is an act of love — for yourself. It's a venue where healing is not just a notion but an experience that develops with each culinary masterpiece.

As you go on this culinary voyage, realize you're not alone. Within these pages, you'll discover a community of tastes and textures that resonate with your journey. Every dish is a testimony to the possibilities of delighting in flavour while supporting your body's drive for homeostasis.

So, flip the page and walk into a universe where ingredients are more than simply things on a shopping list. They're your comrades in the struggle against discomfort, your partners in the dance of health. With the "Rheumatoid Arthritis Diet Cookbook" as your guidance, the kitchen becomes your canvas, and the recipes, your strokes of well-being.

In a world sometimes fraught with obstacles, let this cookbook be your refuge of sustenance — not only for your body but your spirit. Embrace the wonder of tastes, the symphony of healing, and the change a properly planned meal may offer.

Welcome to a domain where health is pleasure, each mouthful is a step towards wholeness, and where the "Rheumatoid Arthritis Diet Cookbook" becomes your valued companion on a path to relishing life, one cuisine at a time.

# CHAPTER ONE

## Understanding Rheumatoid Arthritis

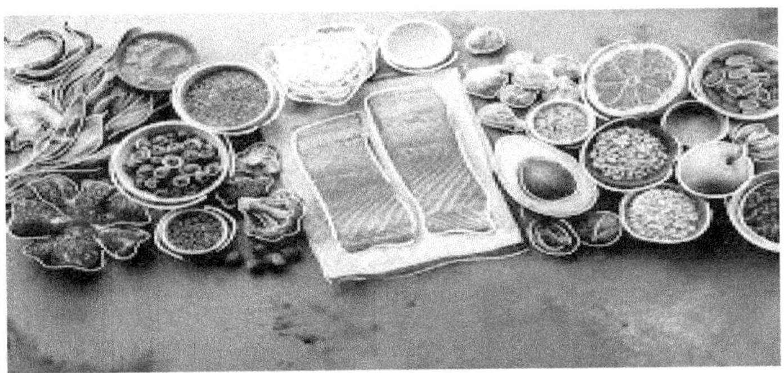

Rheumatoid Arthritis (RA) is a chronic autoimmune condition that primarily affects the joints, producing inflammation, discomfort, and stiffness. Unlike osteoarthritis, which is caused by wear and tear on joint cartilage, RA is characterized by the immune system wrongly targeting healthy joint tissues, leading to joint damage and other health consequences.

**Key topics to learn about Rheumatoid Arthritis include:**

1. **Autoimmune Nature:** RA is an autoimmune illness, which means the body's immune system, responsible for protecting against pathogens, erroneously attacks its tissues. In the case of RA, the immune response primarily targets the synovium—the lining of the membranes surrounding the joints.

2. **Symptoms:** Common symptoms of RA include joint pain, swelling, soreness, and morning stiffness that may continue for hours. The joints most usually afflicted are the hands, wrists, knees, and feet. The condition may also contribute to weariness, poor appetite, and an overall sensation of being sick.

3. **Inflammation:** Inflammation is a hallmark of RA. The immune reaction causes the production of inflammatory chemicals, causing swelling and redness in the afflicted joints. Over time, this inflammation may cause damage to the joint cartilage, bones, and adjacent tissues.

4. **Progression:** RA is a progressive condition that may worsen over time if not effectively controlled. Without adequate therapy, continuous inflammation may lead to joint abnormalities, loss of joint function, and disability.

5. **Diagnosis:** Diagnosis often includes elements, including a patient's medical history, physical examination, blood tests (such as rheumatoid factor and anti-cyclic citrullinated peptide antibodies), and imaging techniques (such as X-rays or ultrasounds).

6. **Therapy:** While there is no cure for RA, numerous therapy techniques seek to control symptoms, decrease disease progression, and improve overall quality of life. These may include treatments like disease-modifying antirheumatic drugs (DMARDs), biologics, and pain relievers. Lifestyle adjustments, physical therapy, and assistive equipment may also be helpful.

7. **Fluctuating Nature:** RA symptoms might alter over time. Periods of heightened disease activity, known as flares, alternate with periods of remission when symptoms lessen or become less severe.

8. **Influence on Daily Life:** RA may significantly influence a person's capacity to conduct daily duties and activities. It may affect one's career, social life, and emotional well-being.

9. **Multisystem Disorder:** RA is not confined to joints; it may also affect other body regions, resulting in inflammation of the heart, lungs, and blood vessels.

Understanding Rheumatoid Arthritis means comprehending the complexity of this autoimmune disorder and the possible obstacles it offers. Effective treatment generally needs a multidisciplinary approach incorporating healthcare specialists, lifestyle alterations, and, as your cookbook recommends, nutritional considerations to help ease symptoms and enhance overall well-being.

## The Role of Diet in Managing Symptoms

Diet plays a crucial part in treating the symptoms of Rheumatoid Arthritis (RA). While nutrition alone cannot cure RA, some foods and dietary choices may help decrease inflammation, relieve pain, and improve overall well-being for persons living with the illness. Here are some crucial aspects to grasp regarding the importance of nutrition in controlling RA symptoms:

1. **Anti-Inflammatory Foods:** Incorporating foods that have natural anti-inflammatory qualities will help lessen the inflammation associated with RA. Examples include fatty fish (high in omega-3 fatty acids), colourful fruits and vegetables, nuts, seeds, and entire grains.

2. **Omega-3 Fatty Acids:** Omega-3 fatty acids, present in fish such as salmon, mackerel, and sardines, have been demonstrated to have anti-inflammatory benefits. These fats help limit the development of inflammatory chemicals in the body.

3. **Antioxidant-Rich Foods:** Antioxidants present in fruits, vegetables, and some spices (like turmeric) might help neutralize free radicals, which lead to inflammation and tissue damage.

4. **Vitamin D:** Adequate vitamin D consumption is crucial for bone health and immune system function. Some studies show that maintaining adequate vitamin D levels may have a favourable influence on RA symptoms.

5. **Calcium:** Calcium is necessary for keeping healthy bones. People with RA may be at a greater risk of osteoporosis due to limited physical activity and corticosteroid medicines. Adequate calcium consumption may assist in promoting bone health.

6. **Plant-Based Proteins:** Incorporating plant-based forms of protein, such as beans, lentils, tofu, and quinoa, may supply necessary nutrients without the saturated fats in specific animal proteins.

7. **Limiting Processed Foods:** Processed foods, heavy in refined sugars and harmful fats, may lead to inflammation and aggravate RA symptoms. It's vital to restrict certain items in the diet.

8. **Gluten Sensitivity:** Some persons with RA may have gluten sensitivity, which may increase inflammation in the body. For people who suspect gluten sensitivity, avoiding gluten-containing meals could be helpful.

9. **Weight Management:** Maintaining a healthy weight is vital for those with RA since excess weight may place further stress on joints. A healthy diet may help weight control and prevent joint pain.

10. **Individualized Approach:** Each person's reaction to dietary modifications might differ. Engaging with a healthcare physician or registered dietitian is vital to designing a personalized nutritional plan that considers unique requirements, preferences, and possible drug interactions.

11. **Hydration:** Staying hydrated is vital for joint health and general well-being. Drinking adequate water may help keep joints lubricated and working correctly.

Incorporating a diet rich in anti-inflammatory foods, antioxidants, and essential nutrients may help to improve RA management and overall quality of life. However, it's vital to highlight that dietary adjustments should complement, not replace, medical therapies given by healthcare specialists. Consulting with a healthcare physician or trained nutritionist is suggested before making substantial nutritional changes.

# CHAPTER TWO

## The Basics of a Rheumatoid Arthritis-Friendly Diet

## Anti-Inflammatory Foods to Embrace

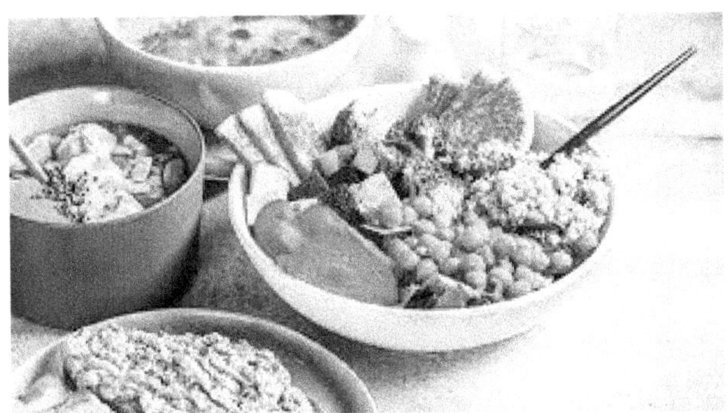

Here's a list of anti-inflammatory foods that patients with Rheumatoid Arthritis may consider integrating into their diet:

1. **Berries:** Blueberries, strawberries, raspberries, and blackberries are rich in antioxidants and have been related to lower inflammation.

2. **Fatty Fish:** Salmon, mackerel, sardines, and trout are abundant in omega-3 fatty acids, which have significant anti-inflammatory qualities.

3. **Leafy Greens:** Spinach, kale, Swiss chard, and collard greens are filled with vitamins, minerals, and antioxidants that battle inflammation.

4. **Turmeric:** This spice includes curcumin, recognized for its potent anti-inflammatory benefits.

5. **Ginger:** Ginger possesses chemicals that may help decrease inflammation and relieve discomfort.

6. **Nuts:** Almonds, walnuts, and other nuts contain healthful fats and antioxidants that assist joint health.

7. **Seeds:** Flaxseeds, chia seeds, and hemp seeds are good sources of omega-3s and fibre.

8. **Colourful Vegetables:** Bell peppers, tomatoes, carrots, and sweet potatoes provide a spectrum of antioxidants and minerals.

9. **Fruits:** Oranges, cherries, and pineapple contain anti-inflammatory chemicals and vitamin C.

10. **Olive Oil:** Extra virgin olive oil includes monounsaturated fats and antioxidants that may help reduce inflammation.

11. **Whole Grains:** Quinoa, brown rice, whole wheat, and oats contain fibre and minerals that promote overall health.

12. **Green Tea:** Rich in polyphenols, green tea has been related to decreased inflammation and better joint health.

13. **Spices:** Aside from turmeric and ginger, other spices like cinnamon and cloves offer anti-inflammatory qualities.

14. **Legumes:** Beans, lentils, and chickpeas are rich plant-based protein and fibre sources.

15. **Cruciferous Vegetables:** Broccoli, cauliflower, and Brussels sprouts are rich in antioxidants and have anti-inflammatory benefits.

Incorporating these anti-inflammatory items into your diet may lead to improved control of Rheumatoid Arthritis symptoms. Remember that individual reactions to meals might vary, so pay attention to how your body responds to various choices and consider working with a healthcare physician or registered dietitian for individualized assistance.

## Foods to Limit or Avoid

Below are some foods that persons with Rheumatoid Arthritis can consider reducing or eliminating in their diet since they might lead to inflammation or aggravate symptoms:

1. **Processed meals:** Highly processed meals frequently include toxic trans fats, refined sugars, and additives that may induce inflammation.

2. **Sugary Snacks and Drinks:** Excess sugar consumption may increase inflammation and lead to weight gain.

3. **Saturated and Trans Fats:** Reducing consumption of fatty cuts of meat, fried meals, and foods rich in trans fats (found in many commercially baked items) might be advantageous.

4. **High-salt Foods:** Excess salt may lead to water retention and could contribute to joint swelling and pain.

5. **Red Meat:** Some research shows that heavy intake of red meat may be connected with increased inflammation.

6. **Dairy Products:** While dairy sensitivity varies, some people find that decreasing dairy may help reduce symptoms.

7. **Gluten:** Some persons with RA can benefit from avoiding gluten-containing foods since gluten sensitivity might increase inflammation.

8. **Nightshade Vegetables:** Certain people could have more significant joint discomfort while ingesting nightshade vegetables, including tomatoes, peppers, and eggplants.

9. **Alcohol:** Excessive alcohol use might induce inflammation and could interfere with medicines.

10. **Refined Grains:** White bread, white rice, and other refined grains lack the nutrients and fibre found in whole grains.

11. **Artificial Trans Fats:** Trans fats, typically present in certain packaged foods and baked products, may increase inflammation and have detrimental health consequences.

12. **Fried Foods:** Fried foods may contain harmful fats and lead to inflammation.

13. **Excessive Omega-6 Fatty Acids:** While omega-6 fatty acids are essential, an imbalance between omega-6 and omega-3 fatty acids might induce inflammation. Limiting sources like some vegetable oils (corn, soybean, sunflower) may be helpful.

14. **Processed Meats:** Processed meats like sausages, hot dogs, and deli meats sometimes include preservatives and chemicals that might lead to inflammation.

15. **Coffee:** Some persons may find that excessive coffee consumption exacerbates RA symptoms. Moderation is crucial.

It's crucial to remember that the influence of these meals might differ from person to person. Keeping a food diary and documenting how foods impact your symptoms might give significant information. A healthcare physician or qualified dietician may provide specialized counselling for your unique requirements and preferences.

# CHAPTER THREE

## Breakfast Delights for Joint Health

### Berry Spinach Smoothie

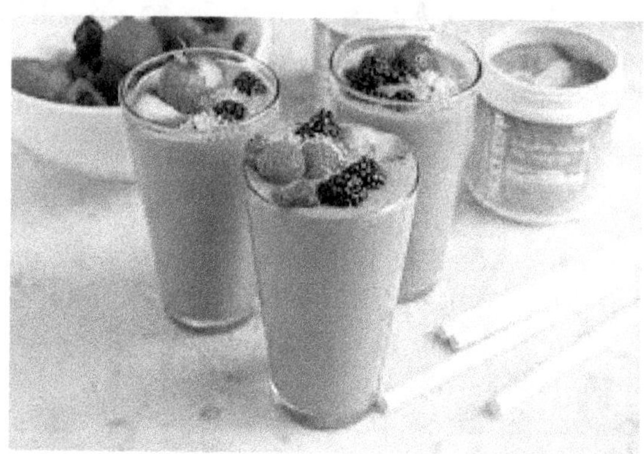

Ingredients:

- 1 cup mixed berries (such as strawberries, blueberries, raspberries)
- One tiny banana
- Handful of fresh spinach leaves
- ½ cup Greek yogurt
- One tablespoon flaxseeds (optional)
- ½ cup almond milk (or any milk of your choice)
- Ice cubes (if wanted)

Instructions:

1. Wash the berries and spinach well.

2.  Peel the banana and split it into bits.

3.  Add mixed berries, banana, spinach, Greek yoghurt, flaxseeds (if using), and almond milk in a blender.

4.  Blend on high speed until the ingredients are fully incorporated, and the smoothie is smooth and creamy. If the mixture is too thick, you may add a bit more almond milk.

5.  If you want your smoothie cooler, add a few ice cubes and mix until they are entirely blended.

6.  Taste and adjust the sweetness if required. Add a drizzle of honey or maple syrup if you want a sweeter smoothie.

7.  Pour the smoothie into a glass and drink immediately!

This Berry Spinach Smoothie is filled with antioxidants, vitamins, and minerals from the berries and spinach. The Greek yoghurt provides protein and creaminess, while flaxseeds contain omega-3 fatty acids and fibre. It's a pleasant and healthy way to start your day, particularly for folks wishing to boost their joint health.

# Chia Seed Banana Pancakes

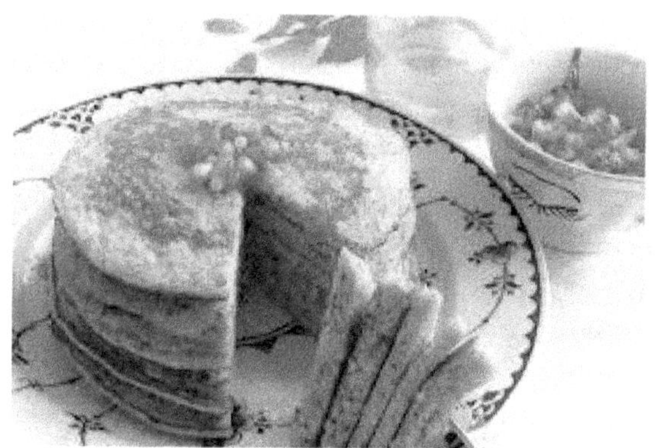



- Two ripe bananas
- Two eggs
- Two teaspoons of chia seeds
- ½ teaspoon vanilla extract
- ¼ teaspoon cinnamon
- Pinch of salt
- Coconut oil or cooking spray for the pan

Instructions:

1. In a mixing bowl, mash the ripe bananas until they are nearly smooth.

2. Add the eggs, chia seeds, vanilla essence, cinnamon, and salt to the mashed bananas. Mix thoroughly until all the ingredients are incorporated.

3. Let the batter rest for around 5-10 minutes to let the chia seeds absorb some liquid and thicken the batter.

4. Preheat a non-stick skillet or griddle over medium heat. You may gently coat the surface with coconut oil or cooking spray.

5. Once the pan is heated, spoon a tiny quantity of the batter onto the pan to make a pancake. You may make them as huge or as little as you desire.

6. Cook the pancakes for 2-3 minutes on one side until you see little bubbles appearing on the surface.

7. Gently turn the pancakes and cook on the other side for 2-3 minutes until both sides are golden brown.

8. Repeat the procedure with the remaining batter, adding extra oil or cooking spray to the pan as required.

9. Once all the pancakes are done, put them on a dish.

Serve the Chia Seed Banana Pancakes warm, and you may top them with more sliced bananas, a drizzle of honey or maple syrup, and a sprinkling of chia seeds for added texture and nutrients. These pancakes are a healthful and gluten-free choice due to the bananas and chia seeds that add natural sweetness and nutrition. Enjoy an excellent breakfast that may help to improve joint health!

# Egg and Avocado Wrap

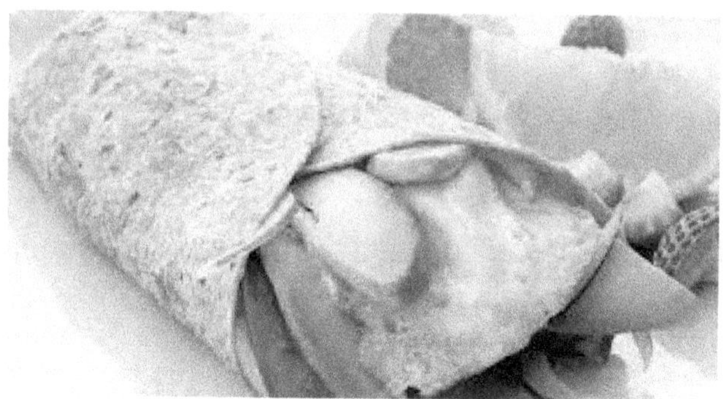



- Two big eggs
- One whole wheat or spinach tortilla
- ½ avocado, sliced
- Handful of young spinach leaves
- Salt & pepper, to taste
- Optional toppings: salsa, spicy sauce, grated cheese

Instructions:

1. Whisk the eggs together in a bowl until thoroughly beaten—season with a touch of salt and pepper.

2. Heat a non-stick skillet over medium heat. Pour the whisked eggs into the pan and heat, gently stirring, until the eggs are scrambled and cooked to your chosen degree of doneness.

3. Warm the tortilla in the pan for a few seconds on each side, or you may wrap it in a moist paper towel and microwave it for 10-15 seconds.

4. Lay the heated tortilla on a clean surface. Place the scrambled eggs down the middle of the tortilla.

5. Layer the sliced avocado and baby spinach leaves on top of the eggs.

6. Add alternative toppings like salsa, spicy sauce, or a sprinkling of shredded cheese if desired.

7. Gently fold in the edges of the tortilla and then roll it up from the bottom to make a wrap.

Serve the Egg and Avocado Wrap immediately. It's a protein-rich, nutrient-packed breakfast choice that gives healthy fats from avocado and critical elements from eggs and spinach. The whole wheat or spinach tortilla provides fibre and enhances the taste. This wrap is tasty and a terrific alternative for folks wishing to maintain their joint health.

## Almond Butter Toast

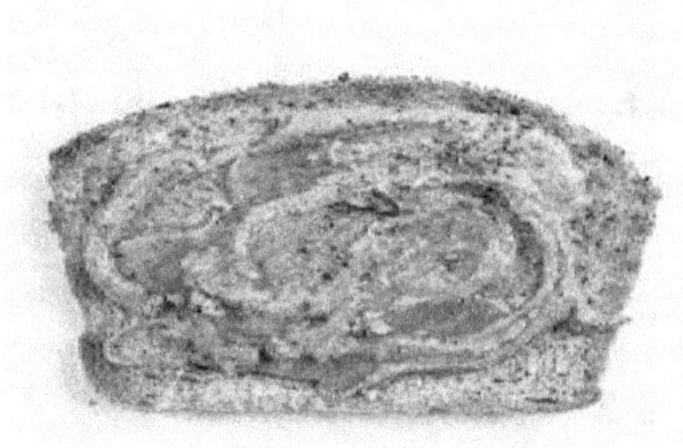

Ingredients:

- Two slices whole grain bread
- Almond butter
- Sliced strawberries or banana (optional)
- Honey or a sprinkle of maple syrup (optional)
- Chia seeds or flaxseeds (optional)

Instructions:

1. Toast the pieces of whole grain bread until they are golden brown and crispy.

2. Once the toast is cooked, put a liberal coating of almond butter on each piece.

3. Top the almond butter with sliced strawberries or bananas for extra flavour and benefits if preferred.

4. For an added touch of taste, sprinkle a tiny quantity of honey or maple syrup over the toppings.

5.  If you'd like, sprinkle chia seeds or flaxseeds on top for extra texture and a dose of omega-3 fatty acids.

Enjoy the Almond Butter Toast as a simple and pleasant morning alternative. Combining whole-grain bread and almond butter gives complex carbs and healthy fats, while the fruit adds natural sweetness and micronutrients. This breakfast pick is tasty and helps joint health and general well-being.

## Turmeric Overnight Oats

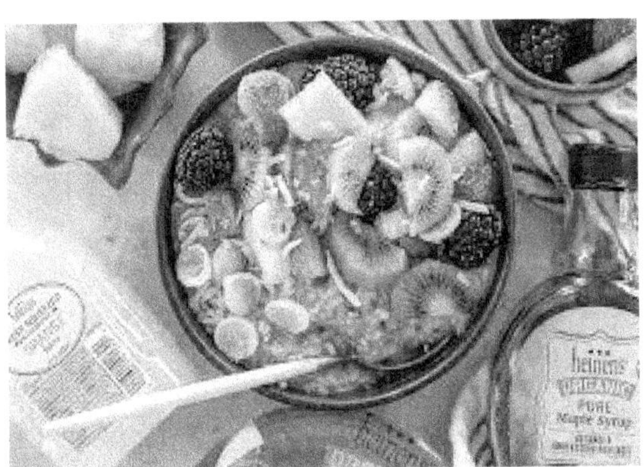

Ingredients:

- ½ cup rolled oats
- 1 cup almond milk (or any milk of your choosing)
- ½ teaspoon ground turmeric
- ¼ teaspoon ground cinnamon
- ¼ teaspoon ground ginger
- Pinch of black pepper (to improve turmeric absorption)
- 1 tbsp chia seeds

- One tablespoon of honey or maple syrup (optional)
- Toppings: Sliced bananas, chopped nuts, dried fruits

Instructions:

1. Mix the rolled oats, almond milk, ground turmeric, cinnamon, ginger, and a sprinkle of black pepper in a jar or container. Stir carefully to ensure the spices are uniformly distributed.

2. Add the chia seeds to the mixture and whisk again. Chia seeds will absorb moisture and help thicken the oats.

3. If you like a sweeter flavour, add a spoonful of honey or maple syrup at this point and combine thoroughly.

4. Close the jar or container with a lid and refrigerate it overnight, or for at least 4-6 hours, to enable the oats to soften and absorb the flavours.

5. In the morning, give the oats a thorough toss. If the mixture is too thick, you may add a splash of almond milk to obtain your preferred consistency.

6. Serve the turmeric overnight oats in a bowl and top with sliced bananas, chopped almonds, and dried fruits for extra texture and nutrients.

Turmeric Overnight Oats give a practical and nutrient-rich breakfast choice. Turmeric is recognized for its anti-inflammatory qualities, and adding black pepper improves the absorption of its active ingredient, curcumin. The oats and chia seeds deliver fibre and energy, while the toppings provide extra vitamins and healthy fats. This breakfast is a terrific option for boosting joint health and well-being.

## Salmon Breakfast Salad

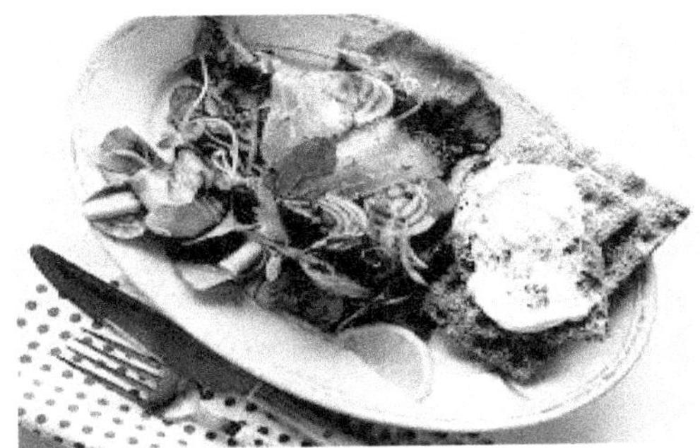

Ingredients:

- 4 oz cooked salmon fillet (grilled, roasted, or poached)
- Mixed greens (such as baby spinach, arugula, or kale)
- Cherry tomatoes, halved
- Sliced Cucumber
- Sliced red onion
- 1 cooked egg, sliced Avocado slices
- Lemon wedges
- Fresh dill or parsley, chopped (for garnish)
- Olive oil and balsamic vinegar (or dressing of your choice)
- Salt & pepper, to taste

1. Prepare the cooked salmon by grilling, baking, or poaching it. Once cooked, let it cool somewhat.

2. In a dish, construct a bed of mixed greens. Arrange cherry tomato halves, Cucumber, and red onion slices on top of the gardens.

3. Flake the cooked salmon into bite-sized pieces and arrange them over the salad.

4. Add slices of cooked egg and avocado to the salad.

5. Squeeze lemon wedges over the salad for a punch of citrus flavour.

6. Drizzle olive oil and balsamic vinegar (or your chosen dressing) over the salad—season with salt and pepper to taste.

7. Garnish the salad with fresh dill or parsley for a splash of colour and freshness.

Enjoy the Salmon Breakfast Salad as a nutrient-packed, protein-rich way to start your day. The combination of salmon's omega-3 fatty acids, mixed greens, and colourful veggies delivers a range of nutrients that enhance joint health and general well-being. It's a pleasant and refreshing breakfast alternative that combines tastes and textures.

# Yogurt and Fruit Parfait

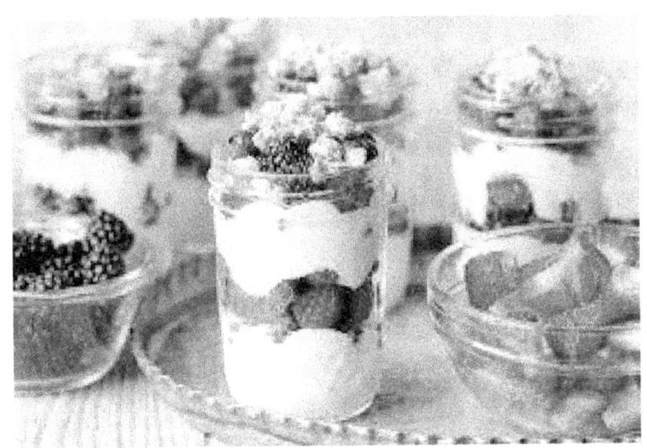

Ingredients:

- 1 cup Greek yoghurt (plain or vanilla)
- Mixed berries (such as blueberries, strawberries, raspberries)
- Sliced banana or other fruits of your choosing
- Granola
- Honey or maple syrup (optional)
- Nuts or seeds (such as almonds, walnuts, chia seeds)
- Fresh mint leaves (for garnish, optional)

Instructions:

1. Start with a tablespoon of Greek yoghurt at the bottom of a glass or a dish.

2. Add a layer of mixed berries, followed by a layer of sliced banana or other fruits of your choosing.

3.  Sprinkle a layer of granola over the fruits. You may also add a drizzle of honey or maple syrup for sweetness.

4.  Repeat the layers until you've used all the components, producing a visually pleasing pattern.

5.  Finish with a dollop of Greek yoghurt on top, and decorate with a few nuts, seeds, and fresh mint leaves if preferred.

Yoghurt & Fruit Parfait is a beautiful, refreshing breakfast choice combining protein, fibre, vitamins, and antioxidants. Greek yoghurt gives protein to keep you satiated, while the fruits add natural sweetness and a range of benefits. Granola gives crunch and added energy. This parfait is tasty and beneficial for joint health and general well-being.

## Green Tea Smoothie

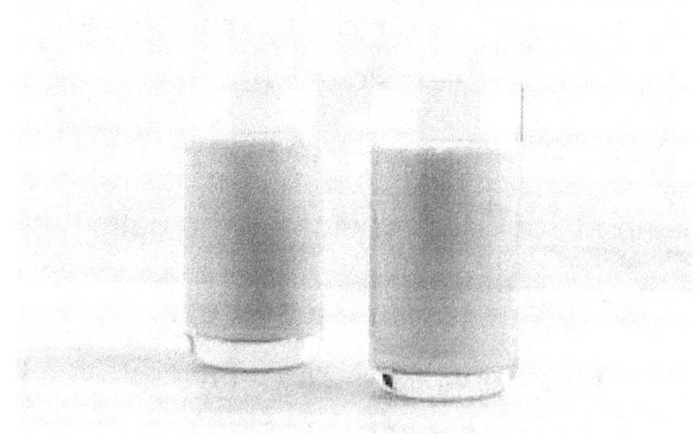

- 1 cup brewed green tea, chilled (you may use decaffeinated if desired)
- One tiny banana
- Handful of spinach leaves
- ½ cup pineapple chunks (fresh or frozen)
- Honey or maple syrup, to taste (optional)
- Ice cubes

Instructions:

1. Brew a cup of green tea to cool to room temperature, or refrigerate until chilled.

2. Mix the cooled green tea, banana, spinach leaves, and pineapple pieces in a blender.

3. Blend quickly until the ingredients are fully incorporated and the smoothie is smooth.

4. If you like a sweeter flavour, add a drizzle of honey or maple syrup and mix again.

5. Add a few ice cubes to the blender and process until they are entirely integrated, and the smoothie is cold.

Pour the Green Tea Smoothie into a glass and drink immediately. This smoothie combines the advantages of green tea, which is high in antioxidants and has possible anti-inflammatory properties, with the vitamins, minerals, and fibre from the banana, spinach, and pineapple. It's a refreshing and healthy way to start your day while boosting joint health and general well-being.


## Coconut Chia Pudding

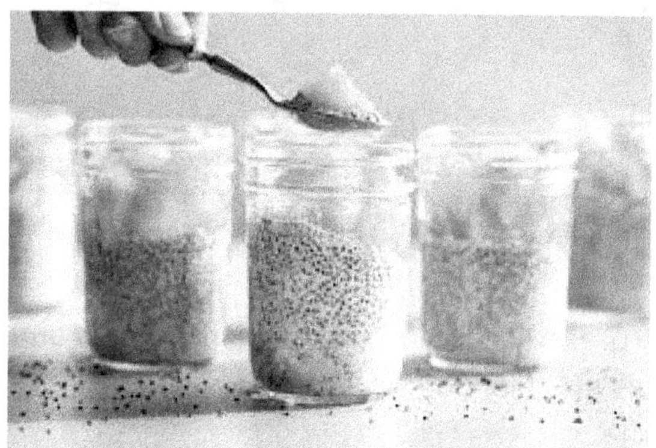

Ingredients:

- ¼ cup chia seeds
- 1 cup coconut milk (canned or carton)
- One tablespoon of honey or maple syrup (modify to taste)
- ½ teaspoon vanilla extract
- Pinch of salt
- Sliced mango or other fruits for topping
- Shredded coconut for garnish

Instructions:

1. Add the chia seeds, coconut milk, honey or maple syrup, vanilla essence, and a sprinkle of salt to a dish.

2. Stir carefully to ensure the chia seeds are appropriately distributed and not clumped together.

3. Cover the bowl with plastic wrap or a cover and refrigerate for at least 4 hours or overnight. This enables the chia seeds to absorb the liquid and thicken the pudding.

4. Before serving, thoroughly stir the chia pudding to ensure it's equally thickened.

5. Spoon the coconut chia pudding into serving glasses or bowls.

6. Top with sliced mango or your favourite fruits.

7. Garnish with a sprinkling of shredded coconut for extra taste and texture.

Enjoy the Coconut Chia Pudding as a creamy and pleasant breakfast alternative. Chia seeds give fibre and healthful fats, while coconut milk provides smoothness and a hint of tropical taste. The natural sweetness of the chia pudding works wonderfully with the freshness of the strawberries. This pudding is tasty and beneficial for joint health and general well-being.

# Baked Sweet Potato with Cottage Cheese

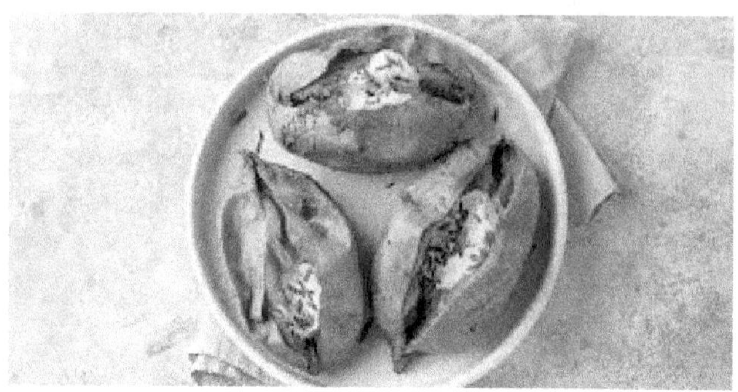

Ingredients:

- One medium sweet potato
- ½ cup low-fat cottage cheese
- Fresh chives or green onions, chopped (for garnish)
- Salt & pepper, to taste

Instructions:

1. Preheat the oven to 400°F (200°C).

2. Wash and clean the sweet potato to eliminate any dirt.

3. Use a fork to poke the sweet potato many times on both sides. This helps steam escape when baking.

4. Place the sweet potato on a baking sheet or the oven rack.

5. Bake the sweet potato in the oven for approximately 40-50 minutes or until it's soft when probed with a fork.

6. Remove the sweet potato from the oven and let it cool slightly.

7. Once the sweet potato is cold enough to handle, create a longitudinal incision on the top, forming a pocket.

8. Gently mash the inside of the sweet potato with a fork to make room for the cottage cheese.

9. Fill the pocket with cottage cheese, allowing it to pour over the edges.

10. Season the filled sweet potato with salt and pepper to taste.

11. Garnish with chopped fresh chives or green onions for extra taste.

Enjoy the Baked Sweet Potato with Cottage Cheese as a pleasant and healthy breakfast alternative. The natural sweetness of the sweet potato blends well with the creamy and protein-rich cottage cheese. This combination includes a balance of complex carbs, protein, and vitamins that help improve joint health and general well-being.

# CHAPTER FOUR

## Nourishing Lunches to Ease Inflammation

### Salmon Salad

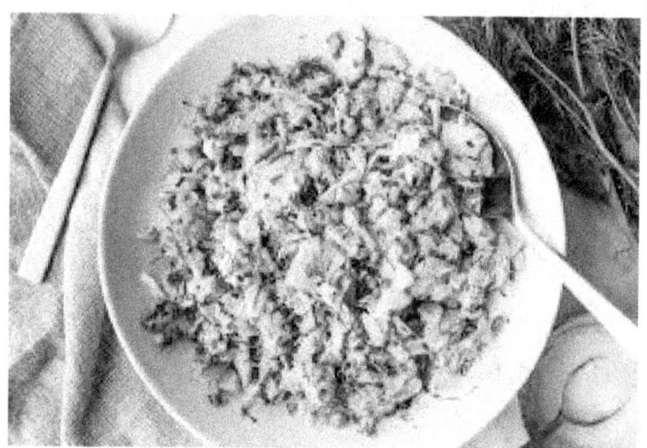

Ingredients:

- 4 oz cooked salmon fillet (grilled, roasted, or poached)
- Mixed greens (such as spinach, arugula, or lettuce)
- Cherry tomatoes, halved
- Sliced Cucumber
- Red onion, thinly sliced Avocado slices
- Nuts or seeds (such as almonds, walnuts, or pumpkin seeds)
- Fresh dill or parsley, chopped (for garnish)
- Olive oil and lemon juice (or dressing of your choice)
- Salt & pepper, to taste

1. Prepare the cooked salmon by grilling, baking, or poaching it. Once cooked, let it cool somewhat.

2. In a big dish, arrange a bed of mixed greens.

3. Arrange cherry tomato halves, sliced Cucumber, red onion, and avocado slices over the greens.

4. Flake the cooked salmon into bite-sized pieces and arrange them over the salad.

5. Sprinkle nuts or seeds over the salad for extra crunch and nutrition.

6. Drizzle olive oil and lemon juice (or your chosen dressing) over the salad—season with salt and pepper to taste.

7. Garnish the salad with chopped fresh dill or parsley for a punch of flavour.

Enjoy the Salmon Salad as a protein-rich and nutrient-packed lunch choice. The combination of salmon's omega-3 fatty acids, mixed greens, and colourful veggies delivers a range of nutrients that enhance joint health and general well-being. This salad is not only tasty but also a refreshing and enjoyable way to enjoy a meal while alleviating inflammation.

# Quinoa with Chickpea Bowl

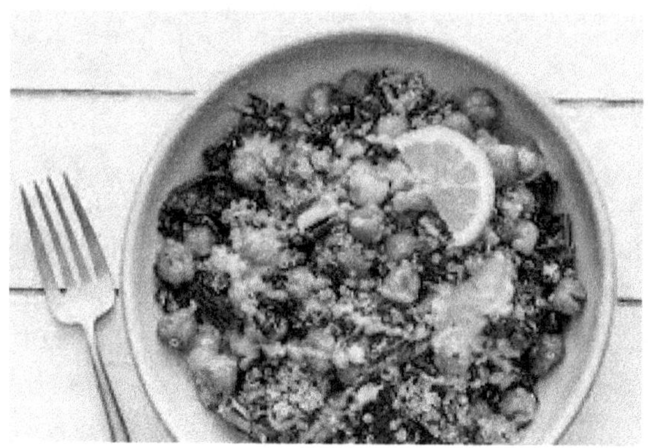

Ingredients:

- 1 cup cooked quinoa
- 1 cup cooked chickpeas (canned or prepared from dry)
- Roasted or steamed veggies (such as broccoli, bell peppers, carrots)
- Sliced avocado
- Fresh herbs (such as parsley or cilantro), chopped Lemon-tahini dressing (follow the directions below)
- Salt & pepper, to taste

Lemon-Tahini Dressing:

- Three tablespoons tahini
- Juice of 1 lemon
- Two tablespoons water
- One tablespoon of olive oil
- One garlic clove, minced
- Salt & pepper, to taste

1. Prepare the quinoa according to the package directions.

2. If using canned chickpeas, drain and rinse them. If using dried chickpeas, make sure they are cooked and drained.

3. Prepare the roasted or steamed veggies. You may roast them in the oven with a sprinkle of olive oil and your favourite spices.

4. In a bowl, arrange the quinoa, chickpeas, and roasted veggies.

5. Add sliced avocado and chopped fresh herbs on top.

6. To prepare the lemon-tahini dressing, whisk together tahini, lemon juice, water, olive oil, chopped garlic, salt, and pepper until smooth and thoroughly mixed. Adjust the consistency with extra water as required.

7. Drizzle the lemon-tahini dressing over the bowl.

8. Season with extra salt and pepper if required.

Enjoy the Quinoa and Chickpea Bowl as a nutritious and satisfying lunch. This bowl is rich with plant-based protein, fibre, and a range of vitamins and minerals from quinoa, chickpeas, and veggies. The lemon-tahini dressing offers a creamy and tart taste to complement the meal. It's a terrific alternative for maintaining joint health and lowering inflammation while having a tasty and enjoyable dinner.

# Turmeric Lentil Soup

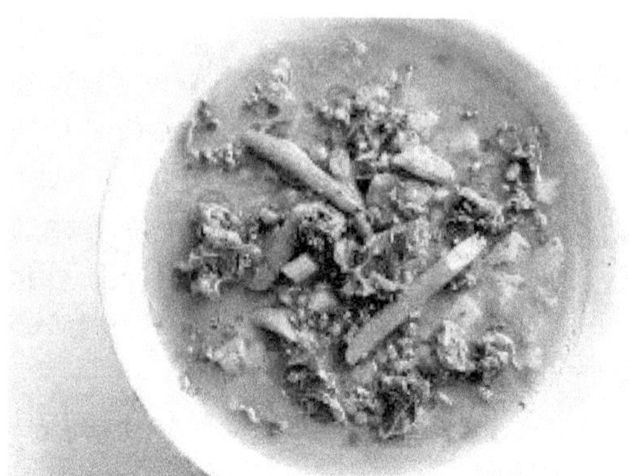

Ingredients:

- 1 cup red lentils, washed and drained
- One onion, chopped two carrots, chopped two celery stalks, chopped three cloves garlic, minced
- One teaspoon of ground turmeric
- ½ teaspoon ground cumin
- ½ teaspoon ground coriander
- ¼ teaspoon ground ginger
- 6 cups veggie broth or water
- One can (14 oz) chopped tomatoes
- Juice of 1 lemon
- Salt & pepper, to taste
- Olive oil, for sautéing
- Fresh cilantro or parsley, chopped (for garnish)

1.  Heat a drizzle of olive oil in a big saucepan over medium heat.

2.  Add chopped onion, carrots, and celery. Sauté for around 5-6 minutes till the veggies start to soften.

3.  Add minced garlic, turmeric, ground cumin, coriander, and ginger. Sauté for another minute until aromatic.

4.  Rinse the red lentils entirely and add them to the saucepan. Stir to coat the lentils with the seasonings.

5.  Pour in the veggie broth or water and add the chopped tomatoes (with their juices).

6.  Bring the soup to a boil, then decrease the heat to low. Cover and let the soup boil for approximately 20-25 minutes or until the lentils are cooked.

7.  Using an immersion or conventional blender, slowly mix the soup until smooth and creamy.

8.  Return the soup to the pot if required. Stir in the lemon juice and season with salt and pepper to taste.

9.  Serve the soup in dishes, topped with chopped fresh cilantro or parsley.

Enjoy the Turmeric Lentil Soup as a warm and anti-inflammatory lunch choice. Turmeric's curcumin is recognized for its possible anti-inflammatory qualities, and this soup blends it with fibre-rich lentils and a combination of veggies and spices. The result is a tasty and substantial soup that helps joint health and general well-being.

## Mediterranean Wrap

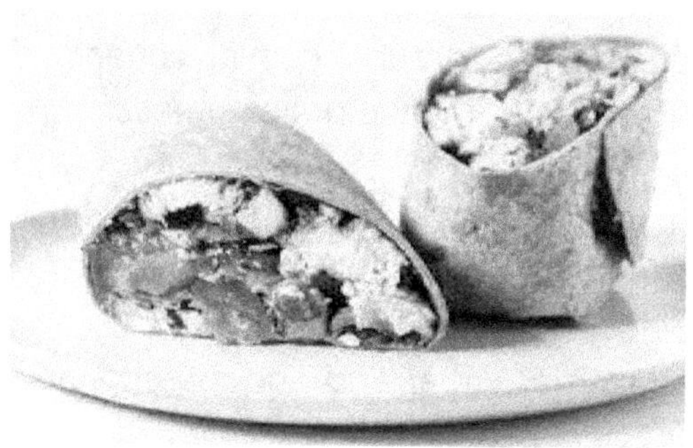

Ingredients:

- One whole-grain or whole-wheat wrap
- Hummus
- Grilled or roasted veggies (such as zucchini, bell peppers, eggplant)
- Kalamata olives, pitted and chopped Feta cheese, crumbled
- Fresh baby spinach or arugula leaves
- Red onion, thinly sliced Olive oil and balsamic vinegar (or dressing of your choice)
- Salt & pepper, to taste

Instructions:

1. Lay the whole-grain wrap on a clean surface.

2. Spread a large quantity of hummus over the wrap, leaving a border around the edges.

3. Place the grilled or roasted veggies over the hummus.

4. Sprinkle chopped Kalamata olives and crumbled feta cheese over the veggies.

5. Add a layer of fresh baby spinach or arugula leaves and finely sliced red onion.

6. Drizzle olive oil and balsamic vinegar (or your chosen dressing) over the ingredients.

7. Season with salt and pepper to taste.

8. Gently fold in the sides of the wrap and then roll it up from the bottom to make a wrap.

Enjoy the Mediterranean Wrap as a tasty and nutrient-packed lunch alternative. This wrap mixes the vivid aromas of the Mediterranean with the nutritional richness of veggies, hummus, olives, and feta cheese. It's a balanced and anti-inflammatory meal option that includes a range of nutrients to help joint health and general well-being.

# Tuna and Avocado Salad

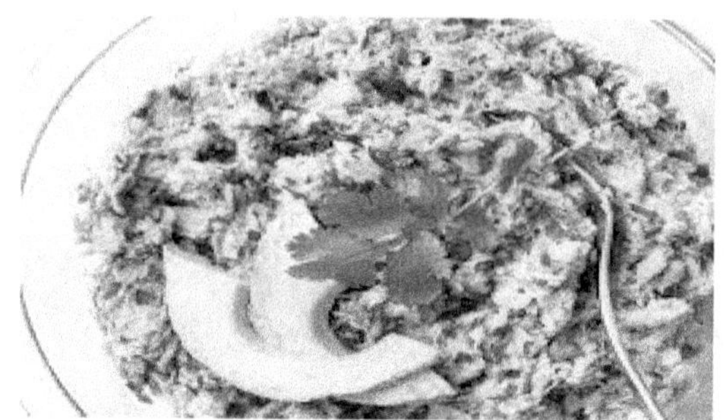

Ingredients:

- One can (5 ounces) tuna, drained and flaked
- One ripe avocado, chopped
- Mixed greens (such as lettuce, spinach, or arugula)
- Cherry tomatoes, halved Red onion, thinly sliced Cucumber, sliced Olive oil and lemon juice (or dressing of your choice)
- Salt & pepper, to taste

Instructions:

1. In a bowl, mix the flakes of tuna and diced avocado.

2. Add mixed greens, cherry tomato halves, red onion, and cucumber slices.

3. Drizzle olive oil and lemon juice (or your chosen dressing) over the salad.

4. Gently mix the ingredients to coat them with the dressing.

5. Season the salad with salt and pepper to taste.

Enjoy the Tuna and Avocado Salad as a protein-rich and healthy lunch choice. Tuna delivers lean protein and omega-3 fatty acids, while avocado adds healthful fats and smoothness. The fresh veggies offer vitamins and minerals, making this salad a pleasant and anti-inflammatory option that improves joint health and general well-being.

## Stir-fried tofu with Veggies

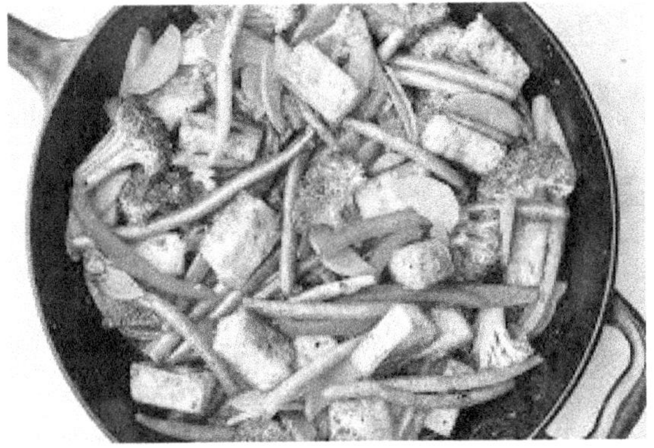

Ingredients:

- 8 ounces firm tofu, diced
- Assorted veggies (such as bell peppers, broccoli, carrots, snow peas)
- Two teaspoons of soy sauce
- One tablespoon of hoisin sauce
- One teaspoon of sesame oil
- One teaspoon of ginger, minced
- Two cloves garlic, minced

- Two teaspoons of vegetable oil
- Sesame seeds, for garnish (optional)
- Green onions, chopped, for garnish (optional)
- Cooked brown rice or quinoa for serving

**Instructions:**

1. Press the tofu to remove the extra water. Wrap the tofu block in a clean kitchen towel or paper towel. Place something heavy (like a plate or a cast-iron pan) on top and set it for approximately 20-30 minutes.

2. Cut the pressed tofu into bite-sized chunks.

3. Whisk together soy sauce, hoisin sauce, sesame oil, minced ginger, and minced garlic to produce the stir-fry sauce in a small bowl.

4. Heat vegetable oil in a big pan or wok over medium-high heat.

5. Add the tofu cubes and fry until brown and slightly crispy on both sides. Remove tofu from the pan and set aside.

6. Add extra oil, if required, in the same skillet and stir-fry the mixed veggies until they are tender-crisp.

7. Return the cooked tofu to the pan and pour the stir-fry sauce over the tofu and veggies.

8.  Stir-fry everything together for another 1-2 minutes until the tofu and veggies are covered with the sauce and cooked.

9.  Serve the stir-fried tofu and vegetables over cooked brown rice or quinoa.

10. Garnish with sesame seeds and chopped green onions, if preferred.

Enjoy the Stir-Fried Tofu with Veggies as a tasty and protein-packed lunch choice. Tofu is a fantastic plant-based source of protein, and when mixed with a range of colourful veggies and a flavorful stir-fry sauce, it produces a filling and healthy dinner. This meal boosts joint health and general well-being, making it a fantastic option for an anti-inflammatory lunch.

## Sweet Potato and Black Bean Bowl

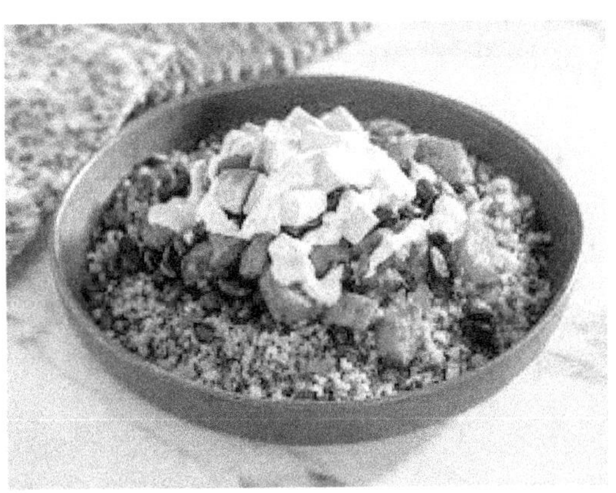

Ingredients:

- One medium sweet potato, cubed one can (15 oz) black beans, drained and rinsed.
- Roasted or steamed veggies (such as bell peppers, zucchini, corn)
- Avocado slices
- Fresh cilantro, chopped Lime wedges
- Olive oil and balsamic vinegar (or dressing of your choice)
- Salt & pepper, to taste

Instructions:

1. Preheat the oven to 400°F (200°C).

2. Toss the diced sweet potato with a drizzle of olive oil and a sprinkling of salt and pepper.

3. Spread the sweet potato cubes on a baking sheet and roast for approximately 20-25 minutes or until soft and slightly caramelized.

4. While the sweet potatoes are roasting, prepare the black beans and veggies.

5. Arrange the roasted sweet potato cubes, black beans, and steamed veggies in a bowl.

6. Add avocado slices and chopped fresh cilantro on top.

7. Drizzle olive oil and balsamic vinegar (or your chosen dressing) over the bowl.

8. Squeeze fresh lime juice over the ingredients.

9. Season with extra salt and pepper if required.

Enjoy the Sweet Potato and Black Bean Bowl as a nutritious lunch choice. The mix of sweet potatoes, black beans, and other veggies offers a balance of complex carbs, protein, and vitamins. The avocado contributes healthful fats and smoothness, while the fresh cilantro and lime juice accentuate the taste. This dish is tasty and a terrific option for maintaining joint health and relieving inflammation.

## Cauliflower and Lentil Curry

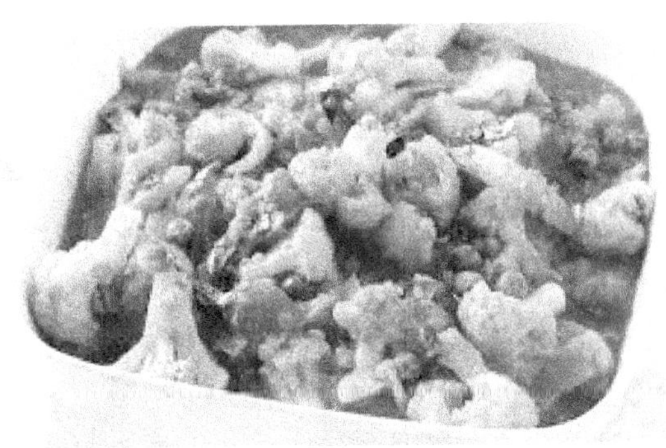

Ingredients:

- 1 cup dry green or brown lentils, washed and drained
- One medium cauliflower, sliced into florets

- One onion, chopped
- Two cloves garlic, minced
- One tablespoon of ginger, minced
- Two teaspoons of curry powder
- One teaspoon of ground turmeric
- One teaspoon of ground cumin
- ½ teaspoon ground coriander
- ¼ teaspoon red pepper flakes (adjust to taste)
- One can (14 oz) chopped tomatoes
- One can (14 oz) coconut milk
- 2 cups vegetable broth
- Juice of 1 lemon
- Salt & pepper, to taste
- Fresh cilantro, chopped (for garnish)
- Cooked brown rice or naan for serving

Instructions:

1. In a big saucepan, heat a dab of oil over medium heat. Add chopped onion and heat until it gets translucent.

2. Add minced garlic and ginger, and sauté for another minute until fragrant.

3. Stir in curry powder, powdered turmeric, ground cumin, coriander, and red pepper flakes. Cook for around 1-2 minutes to toast the seasonings.

4. Add chopped tomatoes (with their liquids) and simmer for a few minutes until the sauce thickens slightly.

5. Add the cauliflower florets and washed lentils to the saucepan.

6. Pour in the coconut milk and vegetable broth. Bring the mixture to a boil, then decrease the heat to low, cover, and let it simmer for approximately 20-25 minutes, or until the lentils and cauliflower are cooked.

7. Stir in the lemon juice and season with salt and pepper to taste.

8. Serve the cauliflower and lentil stew over cooked brown rice or with naan bread.

9. Garnish with chopped fresh cilantro.

Enjoy the Cauliflower and Lentil Curry as a soothing and savoury lunch alternative. This curry mixes the earthy tastes of cauliflower and lentils with fragrant spices and creamy coconut milk. It's a hearty and anti-inflammatory meal that contains plant-based protein, fibre, and essential minerals. Serve it with your choice of grain for a well-balanced meal that improves joint health and general well-being.

# Greek Salad with Grilled Chicken

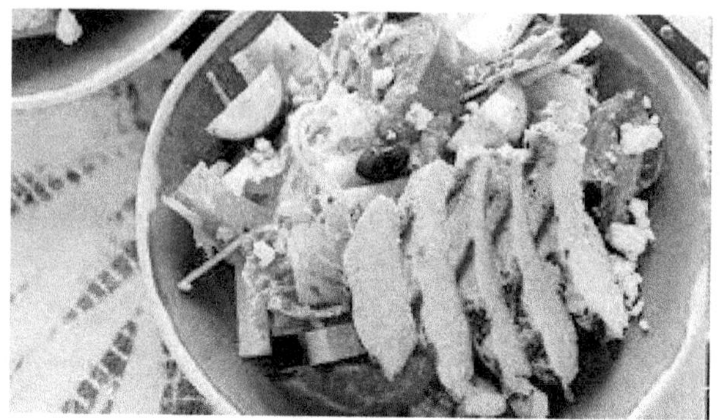

Ingredients:

- Two boneless, skinless chicken breasts
- Mixed greens (such as lettuce, spinach, or arugula)
- Cherry tomatoes, halved Cucumber, sliced Red onion, thinly sliced Kalamata olives, pitted and sliced Feta cheese, crumbled
- Fresh oregano or parsley, chopped Olive oil and red wine vinegar (or dressing of your choice)
- Salt and pepper, to taste. Lemon wedges for serving

Instructions:

1. Preheat the grill or a grill pan over medium-high heat.

2. Season the chicken breasts with salt and pepper. Grill the chicken for approximately 6-8 minutes on each side or until thoroughly cooked, and the internal temperature reaches 165°F (74°C).

3. Once done, take the chicken from the grill and let it rest for a few minutes before slicing.

4. Combine the mixed greens, cherry tomato halves, Cucumber, red onion, and Kalamata olives in a large bowl.

5. Sprinkle crumbled feta cheese over the salad.

6. Top the salad with the sliced grilled chicken.

7. Drizzle olive oil and red wine vinegar (or your chosen dressing) over the salad.

8. Garnish with chopped fresh oregano or parsley for extra taste.

9. Serve the Greek Salad with lemon wedges on the side.

Enjoy the Greek Salad with Grilled Chicken as a fresh and tasty lunch choice. The combination of grilled chicken, mixed greens, colourful veggies, olives, and feta cheese delivers a diversity of tastes and textures. The salad is tasty and rich in vitamins, minerals, and protein, making it a terrific option for supporting joint health and general well-being.

# Zucchini Noodles with Pesto

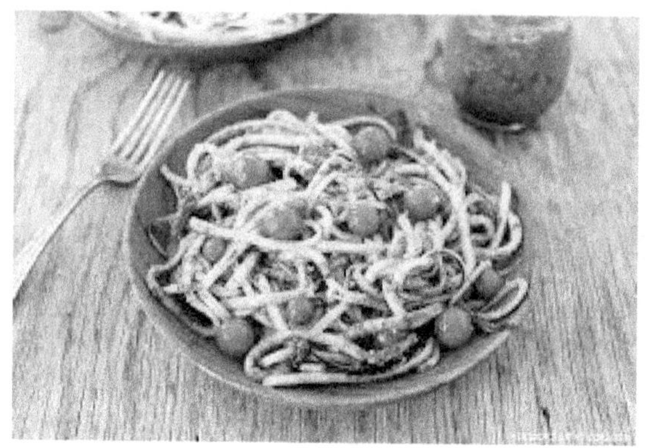

Ingredients:

- Two medium zucchinis
- ½ cup fresh basil leaves
- ¼ cup grated Parmesan cheese 1/4 cup pine nuts or walnuts
- Two cloves garlic
- ¼ cup extra-virgin olive oil
- Salt & pepper, to taste
- Cherry tomatoes, halved (for garnish)
- Grated Parmesan cheese for garnish

Instructions:

1. Using a spiralizer or vegetable peeler, produce zucchini noodles by cutting the zucchini into thin, noodle-like strips. Place the zucchini noodles in a bowl.

2.  Add fresh basil, grated Parmesan cheese, pine nuts or walnuts, and garlic in a food processor. Pulse until the ingredients are coarsely minced.

3.  Carefully sprinkle the olive oil with the food processor running until the pesto reaches your desired consistency. You may need to scrape down the edges of the processor with a spatula.

4.  Season the pesto with salt and pepper to taste.

5.  Toss the zucchini noodles with the pesto until they are fully covered.

6.  Garnish with halved cherry tomatoes and a sprinkling of grated Parmesan cheese.

Enjoy Zucchini Noodles with Pesto as a light and tasty lunch choice. Zucchini noodles give a low-carb alternative to classic pasta, and the homemade basil pesto provides freshness and flavour. This meal is delicious and supportive of joint health and general well-being thanks to its nutrient-rich components.

# CHAPTER FIVE

## Snacks That Soothe

## Greek Yogurt Parfait

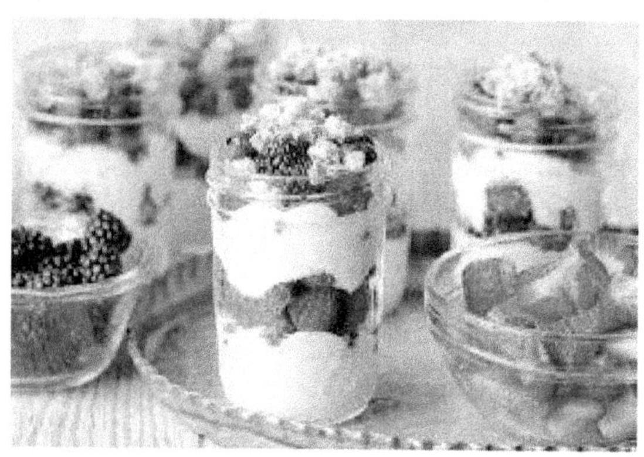

Ingredients:

- 1 cup Greek yoghurt (plain or vanilla)
- One tablespoon of honey or maple syrup
- ¼ cup granola
- ½ cup mixed berries (such as blueberries, strawberries, raspberries)
- Chopped nuts (such as almonds and walnuts) for additional crunch
- Fresh mint leaves (for garnish, optional)

1. Start with a tablespoon of Greek yoghurt at the bottom of a glass or a dish.

2. Drizzle a little honey or maple syrup over the yoghurt for extra sweetness.

3. Sprinkle a layer of granola over the yoghurt.

4. Add a layer of mixed berries on top of the granola.

5. Repeat the layers until you've used all the components, producing a visually pleasing pattern.

6. Finish with a dollop of Greek yoghurt on top and sprinkle with chopped nuts and fresh mint leaves if preferred.

Enjoy the Greek Yogurt Parfait as a delightful and nutrient-rich snack. Greek yoghurt delivers protein and probiotics, while granola adds crunch and energy. The mixed berries have antioxidants and natural sweetness, making this parfait a balanced, calming snack that helps joint health and general well-being.

# Apple Slices with Nut Butter

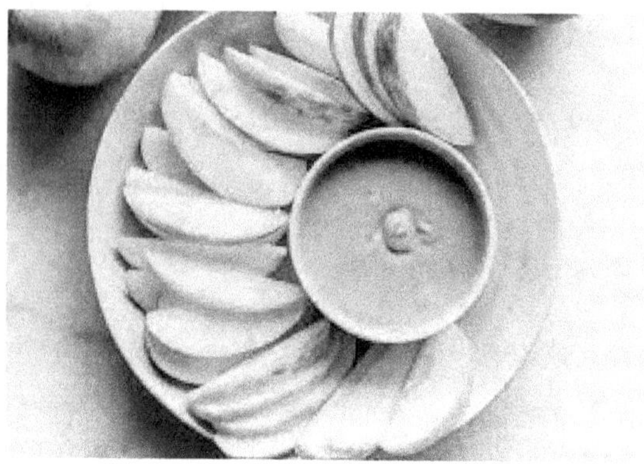

Ingredients:

- One apple (such as Granny Smith, Honeycrisp, or Fuji)
- Nut butter of your choosing (almond butter, peanut butter, etc.)
- **Optional toppings:** sliced almonds, chia seeds, cinnamon

Instructions:

1. Wash and core the apple. Cut it into small slices or wedges.

2. Spread a large quantity of nut butter on each apple slice.

3. Add toppings such as sliced almonds, chia seeds, or a splash of cinnamon over the nut butter if preferred.

4. Arrange the apple slices on a dish or serve them in a small bowl.

Enjoy Apple Slices with Nut Butter as a delightful and healthful snack. Combining sweet and crunchy apple slices with creamy nut butter balances textures and tastes. The beneficial fats and protein in the nut butter and the fibre from the apple make this snack supportive of joint health and general well-being.

## Hummus and Veggie Sticks

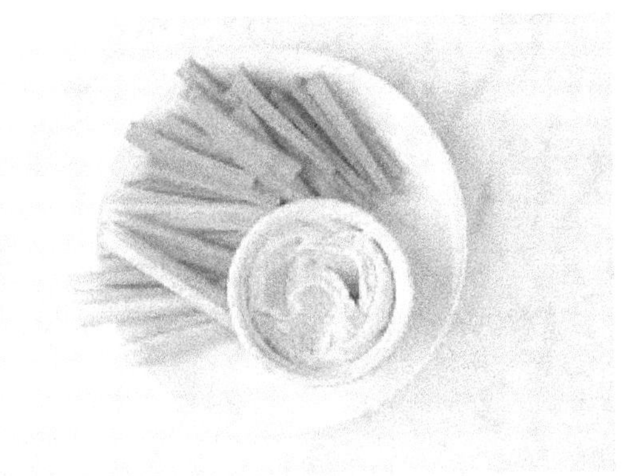

Ingredients:

- Hummus (store-bought or homemade)
- Assorted veggies (carrot sticks, celery sticks, cucumber slices, bell pepper strips)

Instructions:

1. Wash and prepare the veggies by cutting them into sticks, slices, or strips.

2. Arrange the veggie sticks on a platter or in a container.

3.  Serve the hummus with the vegetable sticks as a dip.

Dip the different vegetable sticks into the hummus for a healthy snack. The hummus delivers protein and healthy fats, while the veggies supply vitamins, minerals, and fibre. This snack is tasty and helps joint health and general well-being thanks to its nutrient-rich composition.


## Trail Mix

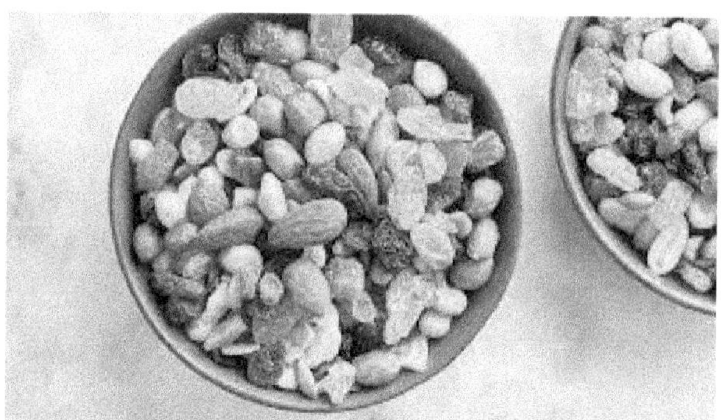

Ingredients:

- Nuts (almonds, cashews, walnuts, etc.)
- Seeds (pumpkin seeds, sunflower seeds)
- Dried fruits (raisins, cranberries, apricots, etc.)
- Dark chocolate chips or chunks (optional)
- Coconut flakes (optional)
- Spices (cinnamon, nutmeg) for taste (optional)

1.  Mix your favourite mix of nuts, seeds, dried fruits, and any extra additions in a dish.

2.  Portion the trail mix into tiny resealable bags or containers for quick grab-and-go snacks.

Enjoy your Trail Mix as a quick and personalized snack. The blend of nuts and seeds delivers healthy fats and protein, while the dried fruits provide natural sweetness and micronutrients. You may adapt the ingredients to your taste and nutritional choices, making this snack supportive of joint health and general well-being. Just remember to enjoy it in moderation owing to its calorie density.

## Oatmeal with Berries

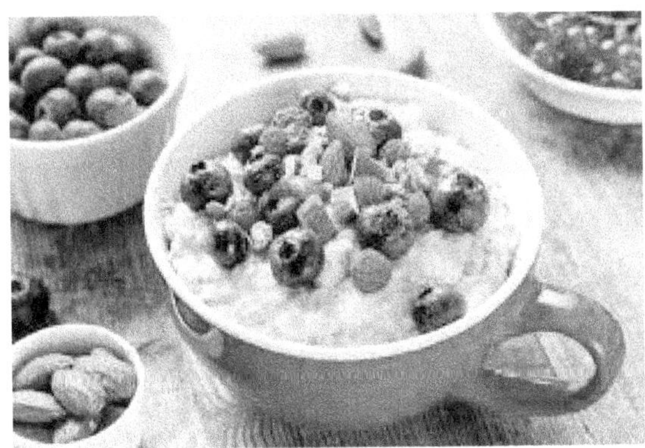

Ingredients:

- ½ cup old-fashioned oats
- 1 cup water or milk (dairy or plant-based)

- Pinch of salt
- Fresh berries (such as blueberries, strawberries, raspberries)
- Honey or maple syrup for sweetness (optional)
- Chopped nuts (such as almonds and walnuts) for extra texture (optional)
- Cinnamon or nutmeg for taste (optional)

Instructions:

1. Mix the oats, water or milk, and a bit of salt in a small saucepan.

2. Bring the mixture to a moderate simmer over medium heat, stirring periodically.

3. Cook the oats for 5-7 minutes or until they reach your preferred consistency.

4. Once the oatmeal is cooked, take it from the heat and let it settle for a minute.

5. Transfer the oats to a bowl and top it with a handful of fresh berries.

6. If preferred, sprinkle honey or maple syrup over the oats for sweetness.

7. Add chopped nuts and a sprinkling of cinnamon or nutmeg for added taste and texture.

Enjoy Oatmeal with Berries as a soothing and healthy snack. Oats are an excellent source of fibre and complex carbs, while berries provide natural sweetness and antioxidants. This snack is soft on the joints and delivers continuous energy, making it a fantastic option for maintaining joint health and general well-being.

## Rice Cakes with Avocado

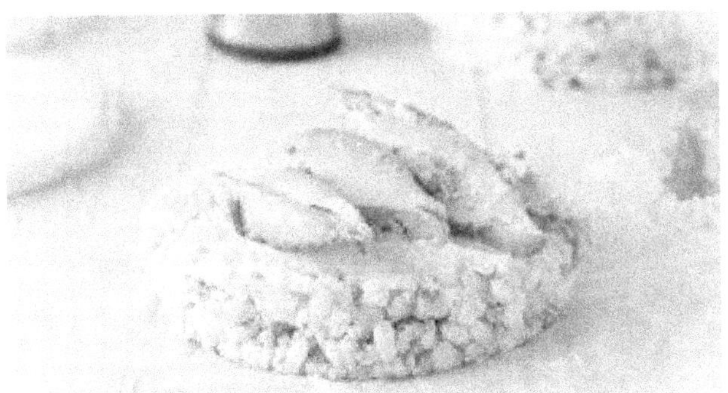

Ingredients:

- Rice cakes
- Ripe avocado
- Sea salt and black pepper, to taste
- Red pepper flakes or spicy sauce (optional, for added taste)

Instructions:

1. Spread a layer of ripe avocado onto a rice cake.

2. Use a fork to mash the avocado onto the rice cake gently.

3. Sprinkle a teaspoon of sea salt and black pepper over the avocado.

4. If you want a little heat, add a sprinkle of red pepper flakes or a splash of hot sauce for added flavour.

Enjoy Rice Cakes with Avocado as a light and pleasant snack. The creamy avocado delivers healthful fats and a spectrum of nutrients, while the rice cake adds crunch and a neutral basis. This simple snack choice may improve joint health and general well-being with its nutrient-rich components.

## Banana with Almond Butter

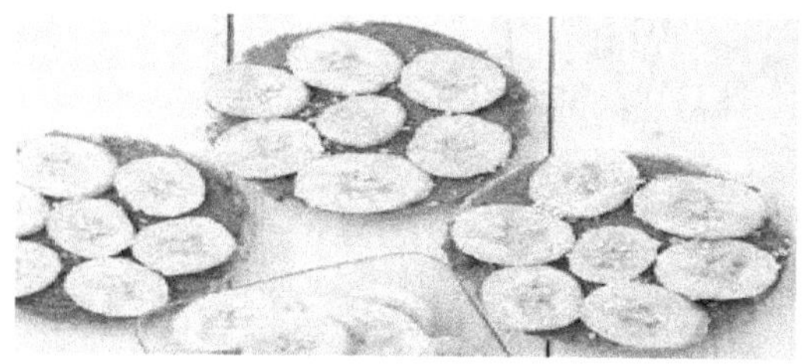

Ingredients:

- ✓ Ripe banana
- ✓ Almond butter.

Instructions:

1. Peel the ripe banana and set it on a dish or in a bowl.

2.  Spread a dab of almond butter over the banana, or dip each banana mouthful into a tiny almond butter dish.

Enjoy Banana with Almond Butter as a delightful and healthy snack. Bananas supply natural sweetness and potassium, while almond butter delivers healthful fats and protein. This combo is tasty and supportive of joint health and general well-being thanks to its nutritional content.

## Cottage Cheese with Pineapple

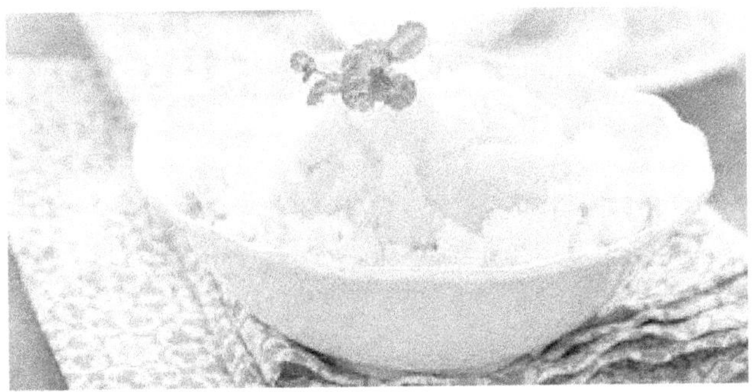

Ingredients:

- Cottage cheese
- Fresh pineapple chunks or canned pineapple nibbles (with 100% juice, drained)

Instructions:

- Place a serving of cottage cheese in a bowl or on a platter.
- Add a liberal piece of fresh pineapple chunks or canned tidbits to the cottage cheese.

Enjoy Cottage Cheese with Pineapple as a simple and delicious snack. Cottage cheese is a fantastic source of protein and calcium, while pineapple adds natural sweetness and vitamin C. This combination is delectable and supports joint health and general well-being owing to its nutritious content.

## Herbal Tea with Nuts

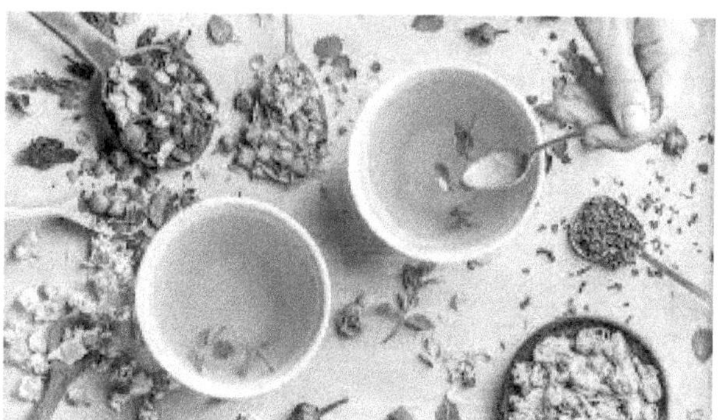

Ingredients:

- Herbal tea bag (chamomile, peppermint, ginger, etc.)
- Mixed nuts (almonds, cashews, walnuts, etc.)

Instructions:

1. Brew a cup of your preferred herbal tea by steeping the tea bag in boiling water for the suggested time.

2. While the tea is steeping, prepare a small handful of mixed nuts.

Enjoy Herbal Tea with Nuts as a peaceful and pleasant snack. Herbal tea gives warmth and comfort, while the mixed nuts deliver healthy fats, protein, and crunch. This mixture is great for a calming respite and may help joint health and general well-being thanks to its nourishing effects.

## Rice Crackers and Tuna

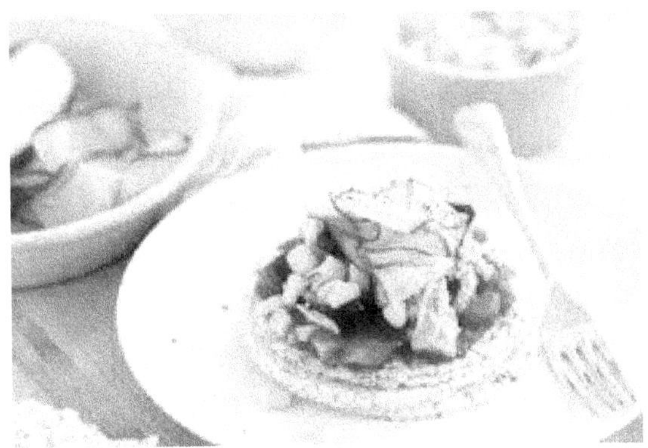

Ingredients:

- Rice crackers (or full-grain crackers of your choice)
- Canned tuna (in water or olive oil), drained Lemon juice
- Fresh herbs (such as parsley or dill), chopped (optional)
- Salt & pepper, to taste

Instructions:

1. Place a portion of rice crackers on a plate or in a container.

2. In a small dish, flake the canned tuna using a fork.

3.  Squeeze a touch of lemon juice over the tuna flakes for extra taste.

4.  If desired, scatter chopped fresh herbs over the tuna.

5.  Season the tuna mixture with salt and pepper to taste.

6.  Serve the tuna mixture beside the rice crackers for dipping or topping.

Enjoy Rice Crackers with Tuna as a protein-rich and tasty snack. Tuna offers lean protein and omega-3 fatty acids, while rice crackers add crunch and a neutral base. This snack choice is handy and may help joint health and general well-being thanks to its nutritious content.

# CHAPTER SIX

## Flavorful Dinners for Rheumatoid Arthritis Relief

## Grilled Salmon with Quinoa and Roasted Vegetables

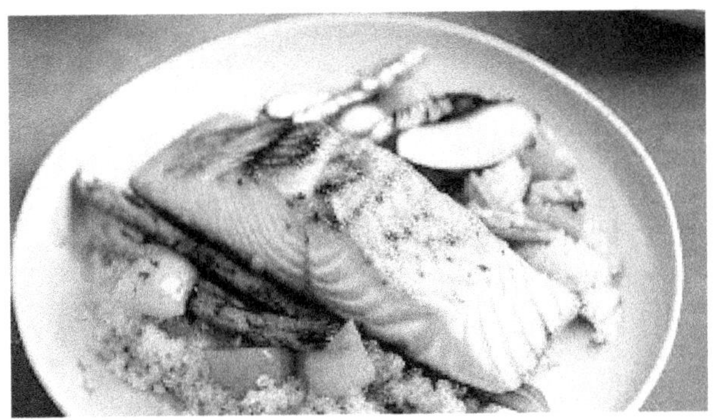

Ingredients:

- Two salmon fillets
- 1 cup quinoa
- Assorted veggies (such as bell peppers, zucchini, broccoli, carrots)
- Olive oil
- Lemon juice
- Fresh herbs (such as dill or parsley), chopped
- Salt & pepper, to taste

Instructions:

1. Preheat the grill to medium-high heat.

2.  Prepare the quinoa according to the package directions.

3.  Wash and cut the different veggies into bite-sized pieces.

4.  Toss the veggies with a sprinkle of olive oil, salt, and pepper. Spread them on a baking sheet and roast in the oven at 400°F (200°C) for approximately 20-25 minutes or until soft and slightly caramelized.

5.  Season the salmon fillets with olive oil, lemon juice, chopped herbs, salt, and pepper.

6.  Grill the salmon fillets on each side for approximately 4-5 minutes or until they're cooked and flake easily with a fork.

7.  Once the quinoa is done, fluff it with a fork and season with olive oil and salt.

8.  Plate the grilled salmon over a bed of prepared quinoa and roasted veggies.

9.  Squeeze extra lemon juice over the meal if desired.

Enjoy Grilled Salmon with Quinoa and Roasted Vegetables as a tasty and nutrient-rich supper. Salmon is a high dose of omega-3 fatty acids, while quinoa supplies protein and complex carbs. The roasted veggies contribute fibre, vitamins, and minerals. This balanced meal helps joint health and general well-being with its anti-inflammatory components.

# Turmeric Chickpea Stew

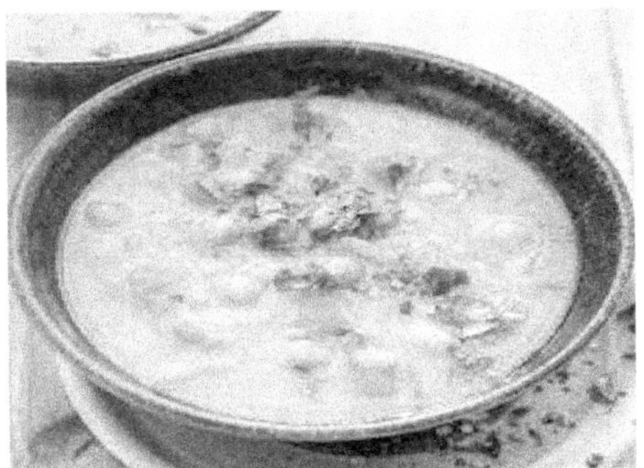

Ingredients:

- One tablespoon of olive oil
- One onion, chopped
- Two cloves garlic, minced
- One teaspoon of ground turmeric
- ½ teaspoon ground cumin
- ½ teaspoon ground coriander
- ¼ teaspoon ground ginger
- ¼ teaspoon red pepper flakes (adjust to taste)
- Two carrots, peeled and sliced
- One red bell pepper, chopped
- One can (15 oz) chickpeas, drained and rinsed
- One can (14 oz) diced tomatoes
- 3 cups vegetable broth 1 cup spinach or kale, chopped
- Juice of 1 lemon
- Salt & pepper, to taste
- Fresh cilantro or parsley, chopped (for garnish)
- Cooked quinoa or rice for serving

1. In a big saucepan, heat olive oil over medium heat.

2. Add chopped onion and sauté until it gets transparent.

3. Stir in minced garlic, turmeric, ground cumin, coriander, ginger, and red pepper flakes. Cook for around 1-2 minutes until aromatic.

4. Add diced carrots and red bell pepper. Sauté for another 5 minutes.

5. Add drained chickpeas, chopped tomatoes (with their liquids), and vegetable broth.

6. Bring the stew to a boil and let it cook for approximately 15-20 minutes to enable the flavours to blend.

7. Stir, add chopped spinach or kale, and simmer until wilted.

8. Squeeze in the juice of one lemon and season with salt and pepper to taste.

9. Serve the stew over cooked quinoa or rice, topped with chopped fresh cilantro or parsley.

Enjoy Turmeric Chickpea Stew as a warming and anti-inflammatory meal. Turmeric's curcumin and the mix of chickpeas, veggies, and spices provide a tasty and nutritious meal that improves joint health and general well-being. Serve it with quinoa or rice for a complete and balanced dinner.

## Mediterranean Grilled Chicken Salad

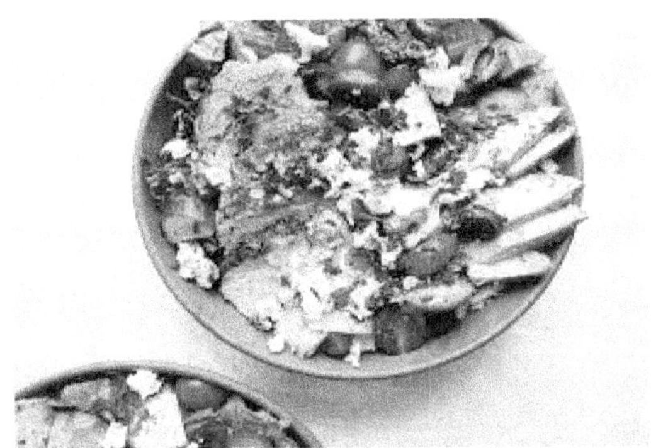

Ingredients:

For the Grilled Chicken:

- Two boneless, skinless chicken breasts
- Olive oil, Lemon juice
- Dried oregano
- Salt & pepper, to taste

For the Salad:

- Mixed greens (such as lettuce, spinach, arugula)
- Cherry tomatoes, halved Cucumber, sliced Red onion, thinly sliced Kalamata olives, pitted and sliced Feta cheese, crumbled.
- Fresh parsley or oregano, chopped Olive oil and balsamic vinegar (or dressing of your choice)

- Salt & pepper, to taste

Instructions:

**For the Grilled Chicken:**
1. Preheat the grill to medium-high heat.

2. Season the chicken breasts with olive oil, lemon juice, dried oregano, salt, and pepper.

3. Grill the chicken for approximately 6-8 minutes on each side or until thoroughly cooked, and the internal temperature reaches 165°F (74°C).

4. Once done, take the chicken from the grill and let it rest for a few minutes before slicing.

**For the Salad:**
1. Combine the mixed greens, cherry tomato halves, Cucumber, red onion, and Kalamata olives in a large bowl.

2. Sprinkle crumbled feta cheese over the salad.

3. Top the salad with the sliced grilled chicken.

4. Drizzle olive oil and balsamic vinegar (or your chosen dressing) over the salad.

5. Garnish with chopped fresh parsley or oregano.

6.  Season with salt and pepper to taste.

Enjoy the Mediterranean Grilled Chicken Salad as a pleasant and savoury meal. This salad mixes the bright aromas of the Mediterranean with grilled chicken, feta cheese, olives, and fresh veggies. It's a well-balanced meal that includes a mix of protein, healthy fats, and vitamins to promote joint health and general well-being.

## Vegetable Stir-Fry with Tofu

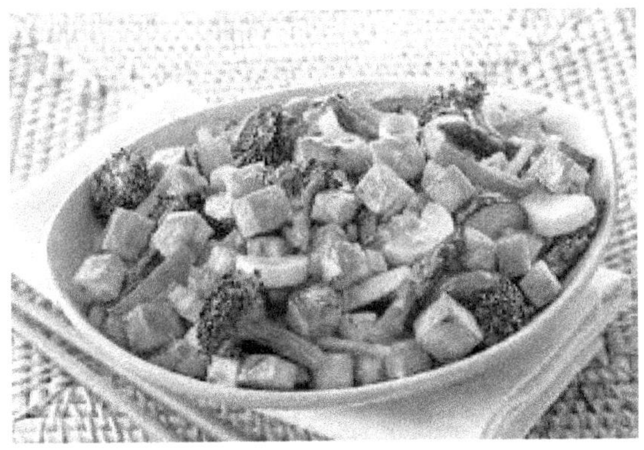

Ingredients:

1.  For the Tofu Marinade:
    - 14 ounces (400g) firm tofu, cubed
    - Two teaspoons of soy sauce
    - One tablespoon of sesame oil
    - One teaspoon of cornstarch or arrowroot powder

2. For the Stir-Fry Sauce:
   - Two teaspoons of soy sauce
   - One tablespoon of hoisin sauce
   - One tablespoon oyster sauce (optional for non-vegetarian version)
   - One teaspoon of rice vinegar
   - One teaspoon of brown sugar or honey
   - ¼ cup veggie broth or water

3. For the Stir-Fry:
   - Assorted veggies (such as bell peppers, broccoli, snap peas, and carrots), sliced two cloves garlic, minced one teaspoon ginger, minced two tablespoons vegetable oil
   - Cooked brown rice or quinoa for serving

Instructions:

1. For the Tofu:
   - In a bowl, combine the marinade ingredients.

   - Add cubed tofu to the marinade and gently toss to coat. Let it marinate for approximately 15-20 minutes.

2. For the Stir-Fry Sauce:
   - Mix the soy sauce, hoisin sauce, oyster sauce (if using), rice vinegar, brown sugar or honey, and vegetable broth in a small bowl. Set aside.

3. **For the Stir-Fry:**

- Heat vegetable oil in a big pan or wok over medium-high heat.

- Add minced garlic and ginger. Sauté for around 30 seconds until aromatic.

- Add the marinated tofu and heat until it's brown and slightly crispy on the edges. Remove tofu from the pan and set aside.

- Add extra oil, if required, in the same skillet and stir-fry the mixed veggies until they are tender-crisp.

- Return the cooked tofu to the pan.

- Pour the stir-fry sauce over the tofu and veggies. Stir-fry everything together for another 1-2 minutes until cooked through.

- Serve the veggie stir-fry over cooked brown rice or quinoa.

Enjoy the Vegetable Stir-Fry with Tofu as a delightful and healthful meal. The mix of tofu, vibrant veggies, and flavorful stir-fry sauce provides a balanced meal that improves joint health and general well-being. The tofu offers plant-based protein, while the veggies supply vitamins, minerals, and fibre.

# Lentil and Vegetable Curry

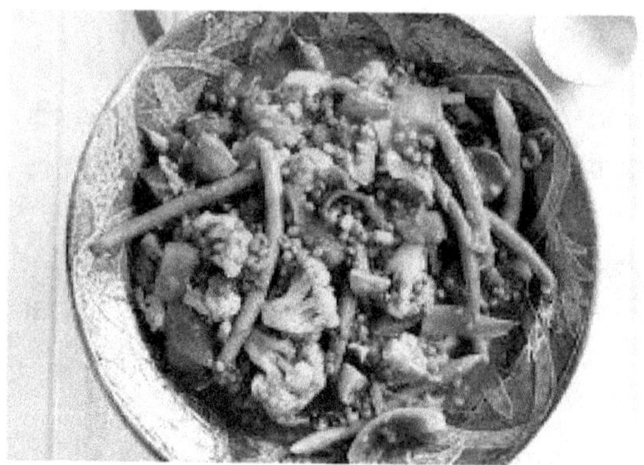

Ingredients:

For the Curry Paste:

- One onion, chopped
- Two cloves garlic, minced
- One tablespoon of ginger, minced
- One tablespoon of curry powder
- One teaspoon of ground turmeric and one teaspoon of ground cumin
- ½ teaspoon ground coriander
- ¼ teaspoon red pepper flakes (adjust to taste)
- Two tablespoons of tomato paste
- Two tablespoons water

For the Curry:

- 1 cup dry green or brown lentils, washed and drained

- Assorted veggies (such as potatoes, carrots, bell peppers), chopped one can (14 oz) diced tomatoes
- One can (14 oz) coconut milk
- 2 cups vegetable broth
- Fresh cilantro, chopped (for garnish)
- Salt & pepper, to taste
- Cooked rice or naan for serving

Instructions:

1. For the Curry Paste:
   - Add chopped onion, minced garlic, ginger, curry powder, ground turmeric, ground cumin, ground coriander, red pepper flakes, tomato paste, and water in a food processor.

   - Process the items until you get a smooth paste. Set aside.

2. For the Curry:

   - In a big saucepan, heat a dab of oil over medium heat.
   - Add the curry paste to the saucepan and boil for a few minutes until aromatic.
   - Add chopped veggies and simmer for approximately 5 minutes, allowing them to soften slightly.
   - Stir in the diced tomatoes (with their liquids) and simmer for a couple of minutes.
   - Add washed lentils, coconut milk, and vegetable broth to the pot. Stir well to mix.

- Bring the mixture to a boil, then decrease the heat to low, cover, and let it simmer for approximately 20-25 minutes, or until the lentils and veggies are cooked.
- Season the curry with salt and pepper to taste.
- Serve the lentil and vegetable stew over cooked rice or with naan bread.
- Garnish with chopped fresh cilantro.

Enjoy the Lentil and Vegetable Curry as a complete and savoury meal. Lentils give protein and fibre, while the diversity of veggies provides vitamins, minerals, and texture. The fragrant spices and creamy coconut milk make this curry a pleasant, anti-inflammatory option that helps joint health and general well-being.

## Zucchini Noodles with Pesto and Grilled Chicken

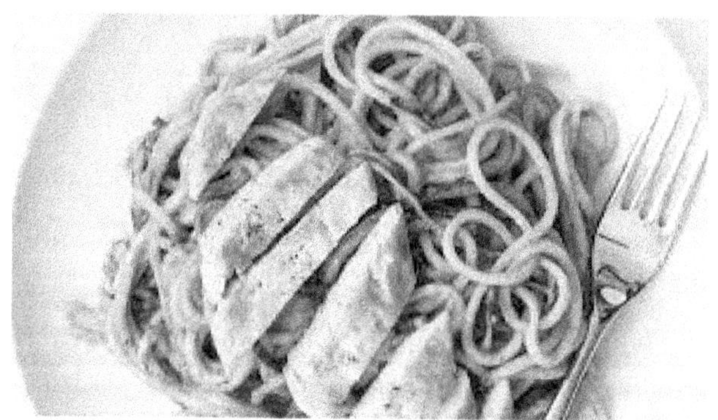

Ingredients:

For the Pesto:

- 2 cups fresh basil leaves, packed

- ½ cup grated Parmesan cheese
- ¼ cup pine nuts or walnuts
- Two cloves garlic
- ½ cup extra-virgin olive oil
- Salt & pepper, to taste

**For the Grilled Chicken:**

- Two boneless, skinless chicken breasts
- Olive oil, Lemon juice
- Salt & pepper, to taste

**For the Zucchini Noodles:**

- 3-4 medium zucchinis
- Salt, to taste

**Instructions:**

1. **For the Pesto:**
   - Add basil, grated Parmesan cheese, pine nuts or walnuts, and garlic in a food processor. Pulse until the ingredients are coarsely minced.
   - Carefully sprinkle the olive oil with the food processor running until the pesto reaches your desired consistency. You may need to scrape down the edges of the processor with a spatula.
   - Season the pesto with salt and pepper to taste. Set aside.

2. **For the Grilled Chicken:**
   - Preheat the grill to medium-high heat.

- Season the chicken breasts with olive oil, lemon juice, salt, and pepper.
- Grill the chicken for approximately 6-8 minutes on each side or until thoroughly cooked, and the internal temperature reaches 165°F (74°C).
- Once done, take the chicken from the grill and let it rest for a few minutes before slicing.

3. For the Zucchini Noodles:
   - Use a spiralizer or a vegetable peeler to form zucchini noodles.
   - Place the zucchini noodles in a strainer, sprinkle with some salt, and rest for approximately 10-15 minutes to absorb excess moisture.
   - Pat the zucchini noodles dry using paper towels before using.

4. To Assemble:
   - Mix the zucchini noodles with the prepared pesto in a large bowl until completely covered.
   - Divide the zucchini noodles among serving dishes.
   - Top the zucchini noodles with sliced grilled chicken.

Enjoy Zucchini Noodles with Pesto and Grilled Chicken as a light and tasty meal. The zucchini noodles have a low-carb basis, the homemade basil pesto provides freshness and flavour, and the grilled chicken delivers protein. This recipe improves joint health and general well-being with its nutrient-rich components.

# Quinoa Stuffed Bell Peppers

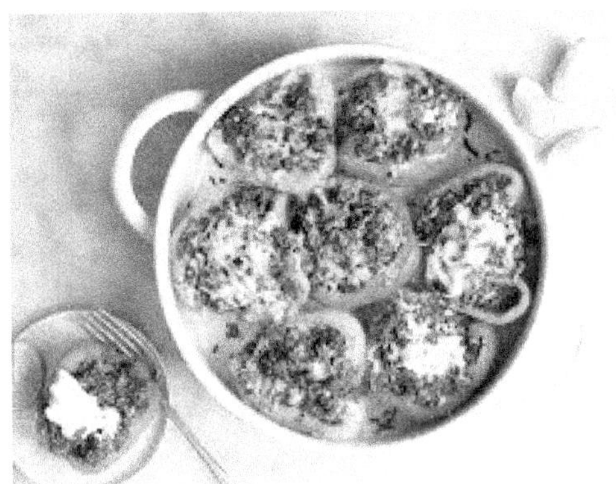

Ingredients:

For the Quinoa:

- 1 cup quinoa, washed and drained
- 2 cups veggie broth or water
- Salt and pepper, to taste.

For the Stuffed Bell Peppers:

- Four big bell peppers (any colour), tops trimmed and seeds removed
- One tablespoon of olive oil
- One onion, chopped
- Two cloves garlic, minced
- One carrot, peeled and coarsely chopped
- One zucchini, coarsely chopped
- One can (14 oz) chopped tomatoes, drained one can (15 oz) black beans, drained and rinsed.

- One teaspoon of ground cumin
- One teaspoon of chilli powder
- Salt & pepper, to taste
- Grated cheese (cheddar, mozzarella, or your preference) for topping (optional)

Instructions:

1. For the Quinoa:
   - Bring the quinoa and vegetable broth (or water) to a boil in a medium saucepan.
   - Reduce the heat to low, cover, and let it simmer for approximately 15-20 minutes, or until the quinoa is cooked and the liquid is absorbed.
   - Fluff the quinoa with a fork and season with salt and pepper. Set aside.

2. For the Stuffed Bell Peppers:
   - Preheat the oven to 375°F (190°C).
   - In a large pan, heat olive oil over medium heat.
   - Add chopped onion and sauté until it gets transparent.
   - Add minced garlic, sliced carrot, and chopped zucchini. Sauté for approximately 5 minutes until the veggies are soft.
   - Stir in drained diced tomatoes, black beans, ground cumin, chilli powder, salt, and pepper. Cook for another 2-3 minutes.
   - Add the cooked quinoa to the veggie mixture and toss to incorporate.

- Fill each bell pepper with the quinoa and veggie mixture, pushing it down slightly.
- Place the filled bell peppers in a baking dish. If using grated cheese, sprinkle it over the tops of the peppers.
- Cover the baking dish with aluminium foil and bake for approximately 25-30 minutes or until the bell peppers are cooked.
- Remove the foil and bake for 5 minutes to melt the cheese (if using).

Enjoy Quinoa Stuffed Bell Peppers as a hearty and healthy meal. The quinoa gives protein and fibre, while the colourful mix of veggies supplies vitamins and minerals. This recipe is not only delectable but also supportive of joint health and general well-being thanks to its nutrient-rich components.

## Baked Sweet Potato with Chickpea Salad

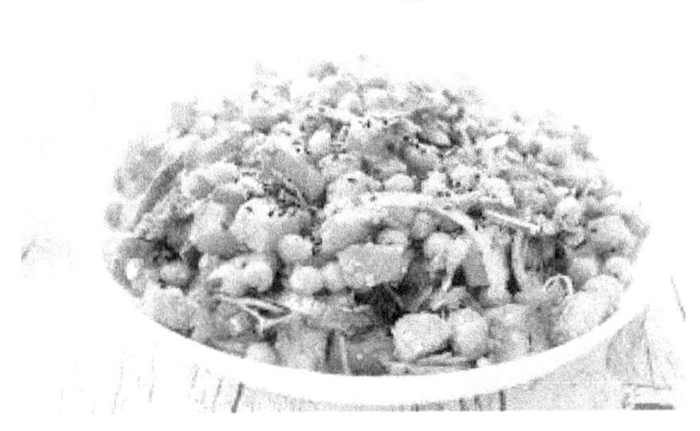

**For the Baked Sweet Potatoes:**

- Two medium sweet potatoes
- Olive oil

Salt and pepper, to taste. For the Chickpea Salad:

- One can (15 oz) chickpeas, drained and rinsed.
- One red bell pepper, diced one cucumber, diced 1/4 red onion, coarsely chopped
- 1/4 cup fresh parsley or cilantro, chopped JuiceJuiceJuice of 1 lemon
- Two tablespoons of olive oil
- Salt & pepper, to taste

Instructions:

1. For the Baked Sweet Potatoes:

- Preheat the oven to 400°F (200°C).
- Wash and clean the sweet potatoes. Pat them dry.
- Rub the sweet potatoes with olive oil and sprinkle with salt and pepper.
- Place the sweet potatoes on a baking sheet and bake for approximately 45-60 minutes, or until they're soft and can be easily punctured with a fork.

- Add drained chickpeas, diced red bell pepper, cucumber, finely sliced red onion, and chopped fresh parsley or cilantro in a bowl.
- Drizzle lemon juice and olive oil over the salad. Toss to blend.
- Season the salad with salt and pepper to taste.



- Once the sweet potatoes are roasted and soft, slice them open lengthwise.
- Use a fork to fluff the insides of the sweet potatoes gently.
- Spoon the prepared chickpea salad over the roasted sweet potatoes.

Enjoy Baked Sweet Potato with Chickpea Salad as a delightful and nutritious meal. The combination of sweet potato and protein-rich chickpea salad provides a well-balanced lunch, promoting joint health and general well-being. The sweet potatoes give complex carbs, while the chickpea salad delivers fibre, vitamins, and minerals.

# Cauliflower Rice Stir-Fry

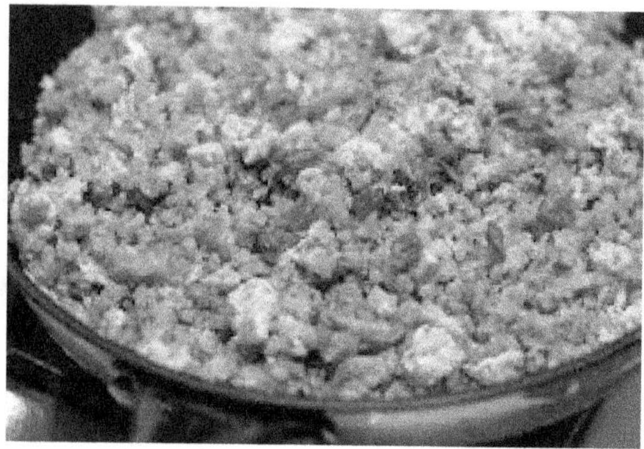

Ingredients:

For the Stir-Fry Sauce:

- Two teaspoons of soy sauce
- One tablespoon oyster sauce (optional for non-vegetarian version)
- One tablespoon of hoisin sauce
- One teaspoon of sesame oil
- One teaspoon of rice vinegar
- ½ teaspoon ginger, minced
- ½ teaspoon garlic, minced
- ¼ teaspoon red pepper flakes (adjust to taste)
- Two tablespoons water

For the Stir-Fry:

- One medium head cauliflower, riced (use a food processor or box grater)

- Assorted veggies (such as bell peppers, broccoli, carrots), sliced 1 cup cooked protein (tofu, chicken, shrimp, etc.), diced (optional)
- Two teaspoons of vegetable oil
- Two eggs, beaten (optional for non-vegetarian version)
- Green onions, chopped (for garnish)
- Sesame seeds (for garnish)

Instructions:

1. For the Stir-Fry Sauce:
   - Mix soy sauce, oyster sauce (if using), hoisin sauce, sesame oil, rice vinegar, minced ginger, minced garlic, red pepper flakes, and water in a small bowl. Set aside.

2. For the Stir-Fry:
   - In a big pan or wok, heat vegetable oil over medium-high heat.
   - If using eggs, press the veggies to the side of the pan and pour the beaten eggs into the vacant area. Scramble the eggs until cooked through, then combine them with the veggies.
   - Add the varied cut veggies to the skillet and stir-fry for a few minutes until they soften.
   - Add cooked protein to the pan and stir-fry for another minute to heat it through.
   - Add the riced cauliflower to the pan and stir-fry for approximately 2-3 minutes until the cauliflower is soft and hot.

- Pour the stir-fry sauce over the items in the pan. Stir-fry everything together to coat with the sauce evenly.
- Garnish with chopped green onions and sesame seeds.

Enjoy Cauliflower Rice Stir-Fry as a low-carb and tasty meal. The cauliflower rice offers health benefits, while the variety of veggies and optional protein gives texture and diversity. This recipe improves joint health and well-being with nutrient-rich ingredients and balanced tastes.

## Greek-style Lentil Salad

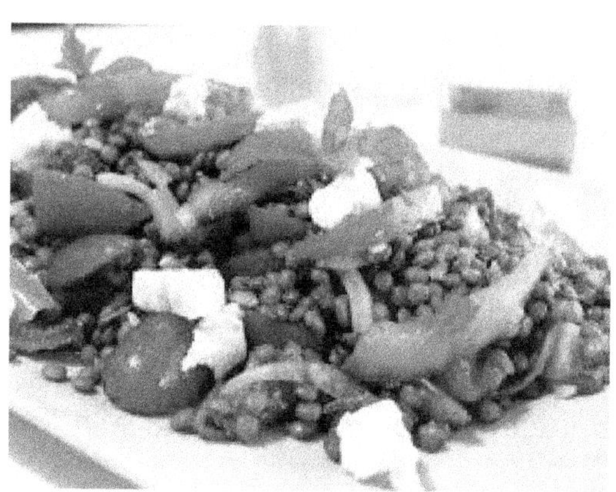

Ingredients:

For the Lentils:
- 1 cup dry green or brown lentils, washed and drained
- 3 cups of water or vegetable broth
- Salt, to taste

- One cucumber diced one red bell pepper, diced one red onion, coarsely chopped
- 1 cup cherry tomatoes, halved 1/2 cup Kalamata olives, pitted and sliced
- ½ cup crumbled feta cheese
- Fresh parsley, chopped
- Fresh mint, chopped (optional)
- Juice of 1 lemon
- Three tablespoons extra-virgin olive oil
- Salt & pepper, to taste

Instructions:

1. For the Lentils:

- Bring the lentils and water (or veggie broth) to a boil in a medium saucepan.
- Reduce the heat to low, cover, and allow the lentils to simmer for approximately 20-25 minutes or until soft but not mushy.
- Drain any excess water and season the lentils with a pinch of salt. Set aside.

2. For the Salad:

- Add the cooked lentils, diced cucumber, red bell pepper, finely chopped red onion, cherry tomato halves, sliced Kalamata olives, and crumbled feta cheese in a large bowl.

- Mix the lemon juice and extra-virgin olive oil in a small bowl to produce the dressing.
- Drizzle the dressing over the salad components and mix everything.
- Add chopped fresh parsley and mint (if used) to the salad. Gently mix to blend.
- Season the salad with salt and pepper to taste.

Enjoy Greek-style Lentil Salad as a pleasant and healthy meal. Lentils give protein and fibre, while the array of veggies, olives, and feta cheese provides colourful tastes and textures. This salad is tasty and supportive of joint health and general well-being thanks to its nutrient-rich components.

# CHAPTER SEVEN

## Sides and Sustenance

## Steamed Broccoli

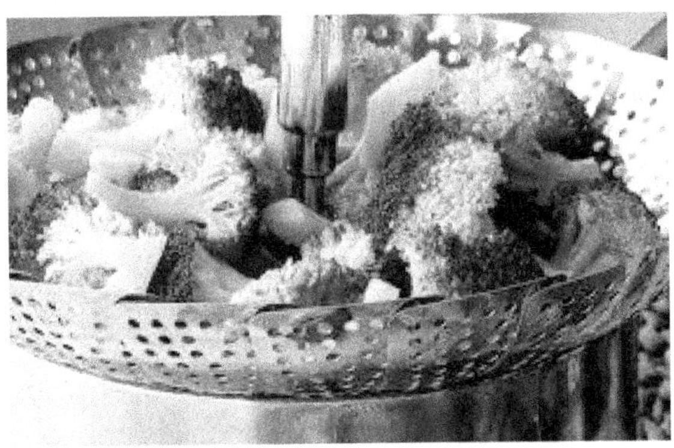

Ingredients:

- Fresh broccoli florets
- Water Salt (optional)

Instructions:

1. Prepare the Broccoli:
   - Wash the broccoli florets well under cold water.
   - If the stems are thick, peel them with a vegetable peeler to remove rough outer layers.
   - Cut the broccoli into bite-sized florets.

2. Set Up a Steamer:

**Stovetop Steaming:**
- Place a steamer basket inside a saucepan.
- Fill the pot with approximately an inch of water, ensuring the water level is below the steamer basket.
- Bring the water to a boil.
- Microwave Steaming: Place the broccoli florets in a microwave-safe dish. Add a spoonful of water to the plate.

3. Steam the Broccoli:

**Stovetop Steaming:**
- Place the broccoli florets in the steamer basket.
- Cover the saucepan with a cover and steam for approximately 3-5 minutes or until the broccoli is cooked.
- Check the broccoli with a fork — it should pierce easily, but the florets should still be slightly firm.
- Microwave Steaming: Cover the microwave-safe dish with a microwave-safe plate or plastic wrap. Microwave on high for approximately 2-4 minutes, checking for doneness after 2 minutes.

4. Season and Serve:
- Once the broccoli is cooked to your chosen degree of softness, take it from the steamer.
- If desired, sprinkle salt over the cooked broccoli for an extra taste.

Steamed broccoli is a healthy, flexible side dish that may complement several entrees. It's rich in vitamins, minerals, and antioxidants, making it a terrific option to promote joint health and general well-being.

## Mixed Berry Salad

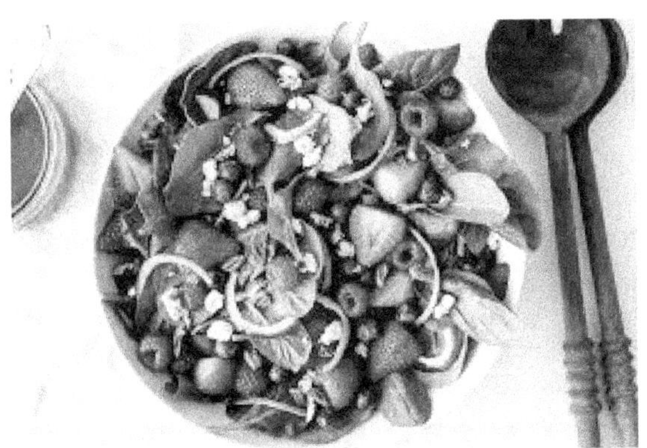

Ingredients:

For the Salad:

- Mixed berries (blueberries, strawberries, raspberries, blackberries) Fresh mint leaves, diced (optional) For the

Dressing:

- Juice of 1 lemon
- Two tablespoons of honey or maple syrup
- One teaspoon of balsamic vinegar (optional)
- Fresh mint leaves, chopped (optional)

1. **For the Salad:**

   - **Wash the Berries:** Rinse the berries under cold water and carefully pat them dry using paper towels. If using strawberries, remove the stems and slice them.

   - **Blend Berries:** In a mixing dish, blend the mixed berries. You may use equal portions of each variety or vary your desired quantities.

   - **Add Mint (Optional):** If using fresh mint leaves, cut them and add them to the mixed berries. Mint lends a pleasant flavour to the salad.

2. **For the Dressing:**

   - **Prepare the Dressing:** In a small bowl, mix the lemon juice, honey or maple syrup, and balsamic vinegar (if using). The balsamic vinegar provides a delicate depth of flavour to the dressing.

   - **Add Mint (Optional):** If preferred, add chopped mint leaves to the dressing and give it a little swirl.

3. **To Assemble:**

   - **Drizzle Dressing:** Pour the dressing over the mixed berries in the bowl.

- **Gently Toss:** Using a spoon or your hands, gently toss the berries to coat them equally with the dressing.

- **Serve:** Transfer the mixed berry salad to serving dishes or platters. Garnish with more mint leaves if desired.

Enjoy the Mixed Berry Salad as a refreshing, antioxidant-rich side supporting joint health and general well-being. The mix of vivid berries and the spicy, somewhat sweet dressing makes this salad a lovely complement to any dinner.

## Quinoa Pilaf

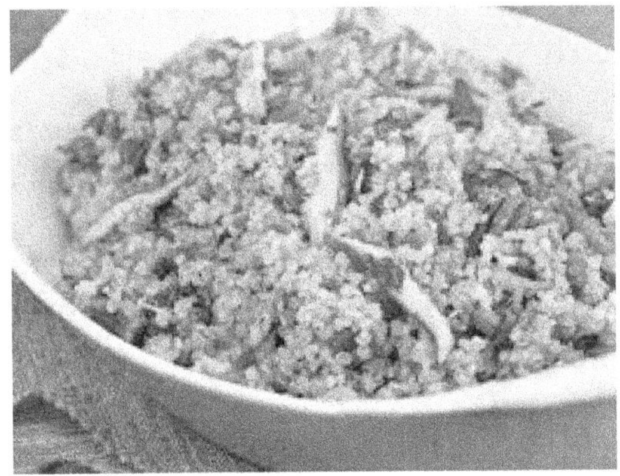

Ingredients:

- 1 cup quinoa, washed and drained
- 2 cups veggie broth or water
- One tablespoon of olive oil or butter
- One small onion, coarsely chopped

- Two cloves garlic, minced
- ½ cup chopped veggies (carrots, bell peppers, peas, etc.)
- ¼ cup chopped nuts (almonds, cashews, etc.)
- ¼ cup dried fruit (raisins, cranberries, apricots, etc.)
- Salt & pepper, to taste
- Fresh herbs (such as parsley, thyme, or cilantro), chopped (optional)

Instructions:

1. **Prepare Quinoa:**
   - Bring the quinoa and vegetable broth (or water) to a boil in a medium saucepan.
   - Reduce the heat to low, cover, and let it simmer for approximately 15-20 minutes, or until the quinoa is cooked and the liquid is absorbed.
   - Fluff the quinoa with a fork.

2. **Sauté Onion and Garlic:** Heat olive oil or butter over medium heat in a large pan. Add finely chopped onion and sauté until it gets transparent.

3. Add veggies: Add the minced garlic and chopped veggies to the pan. Sauté for around 3-5 minutes until the veggies are soft.

4. **Combine Quinoa:** Add the cooked quinoa to the pan with the sautéed veggies. Stir to blend and let the flavours mingle for a couple of minutes.

5. **Add Nuts and Dried Fruit:** Mix the chopped nuts and dried fruit. This adds structure and a hint of sweetness to the pilaf.

6. **Season:** Season the quinoa pilaf with salt and pepper to taste. Be wary of the salt if your vegetable soup is already seasoned.

7. **Garnish with Herbs:** Scatter chopped fresh herbs over the quinoa pilaf right before serving. This provides an additional layer of taste.

8. **Serve:** Transfer the quinoa pilaf to a serving dish and enjoy it as a tasty and nutrient-rich side dish.

Quinoa pilaf is a flexible and nutritional meal that delivers protein and complex carbs, making it a perfect addition to promote joint health and general well-being. You may alter the veggies, nuts, and dried fruits for a tasty and balanced dinner.

## Roasted Sweet Potatoes

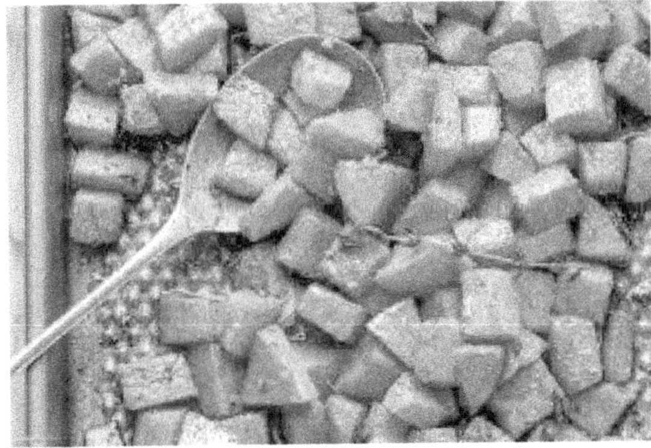

- Sweet potatoes
- Olive oil
- Salt & pepper, to taste
- **Optional seasonings:** cinnamon, paprika, thyme, rosemary, etc.



1. **Preheat the Oven:** Preheat the oven to 400°F (200°C).

2. **Prepare the Sweet Potatoes:** Wash and clean the sweet potatoes to eliminate any dirt. You may peel them if preferred, but keeping the skin on gives additional nutrients and taste.

3. **Cut into Pieces:** Cut the sweet potatoes into bite-sized cubes or wedges. Make sure the pieces are around the same size to achieve consistent frying.

4. **Toss with Olive Oil:** In a mixing dish, toss the sweet potato pieces with olive oil. The oil helps the sweet potatoes grow crispy while roasting.

5. **Season:** Sprinkle salt and pepper over the sweet potatoes, and feel free to add any other ingredients, like cinnamon for sweetness or paprika for a hint of smokiness.

6. **Spread on Baking Sheet:** Spread the seasoned sweet potato pieces in a single layer on a baking sheet. You may line the baking sheet with parchment paper for easier cleaning.

7. **Cook in the Oven:** Place the baking sheet in the oven and cook for around 25-30 minutes. Check and toss the sweet potatoes halfway through to ensure uniform cooking and browning.

8. **Check for Doneness:** The sweet potatoes are done when they are soft on the inside and crispy on the exterior. Pierce them with a fork to check for doneness.

9. **Serve:** Remove the sweet potatoes from the oven once roasted to your preferred degree of softness. Transfer them to a serving plate and enjoy.

Roasted sweet potatoes are a delightful and nutrient-rich side dish that may enhance joint health and general well-being. They offer complex carbs, fibre, and vitamins. Feel free to tweak the spices to your taste preferences for a tasty touch to your meals.

## Cauliflower Mash

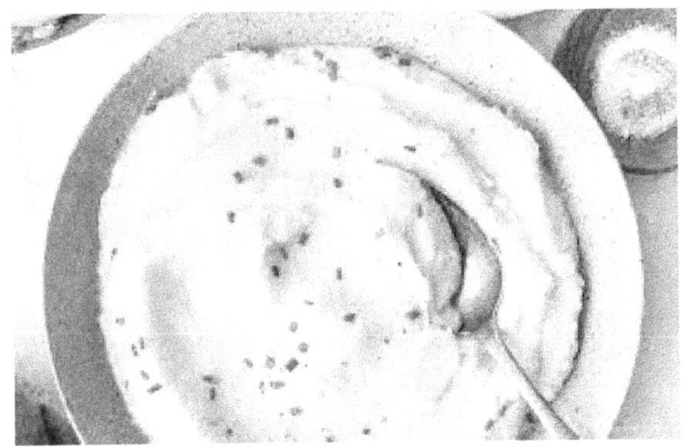

- One medium-head cauliflower, cleaned and cut into florets
- Two cloves garlic peeled
- Two tablespoons of butter or olive oil
- ¼ cup milk or milk substitute (such as almond milk)
- Salt & pepper, to taste
- Optional add-ins: grated Parmesan cheese, chopped fresh herbs (chives, parsley), roasted garlic, nutritional yeast

Instructions:

1. **Steam the Cauliflower:** Place the cauliflower florets and peeled garlic cloves in a steamer basket. Steam for approximately 10-12 minutes or until the cauliflower is exceptionally soft and easily punctured with a fork.

2. **Drain and Pat Dry:** Once the cauliflower is done, take it from the steamer and set it on a clean kitchen towel or paper towel to absorb extra moisture. This step is necessary to prevent the cauliflower mash from becoming watery.

3. **Mash the Cauliflower:** Combine the steamed cauliflower and garlic in a food processor or blender. Pulse a few times to break it down.

4. **Add Butter/Oil and Milk:**
   - Add the butter or olive oil and a splash of milk to the food processor.

- Blend until the mixture is smooth and creamy. You may need to scrape along the edges of the processor to ensure everything is properly blended.
- Adjust the quantity of milk for your desired consistency.

5. **Season and Customize:** Season the cauliflower mash with salt and pepper to taste. Add grated Parmesan cheese, minced fresh herbs, roasted garlic, or nutritional yeast for extra taste if preferred.

6. **Adjust Consistency:** If the mash is too thick, you may add a bit more milk and combine again. If it's too thin, heat it gently on the burner to evaporate some of the liquid.

7. **Serve:** Transfer the cauliflower mash to a serving plate and top with more herbs or a drizzle of olive oil if preferred.

Cauliflower mash is a nutrient-rich and lower-carb alternative to mashed potatoes. It delivers vitamins, fibre, and antioxidants, boosting joint health and general well-being. Customize the taste and texture to your desire for a pleasant and healthful side dish.

# Garlic Sauteed Spinach

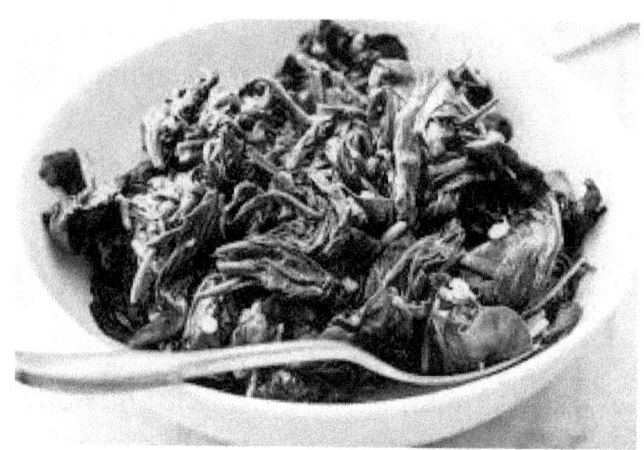

Ingredients:

- Fresh spinach leaves, cleaned and dried
- Olive oil
- Garlic cloves, minced
- Salt & pepper, to taste
- **Optional additions:** red pepper flakes, lemon zest, roasted pine nuts

Instructions:

1. **Prepare the Spinach:** Wash the spinach leaves well and dry them with a kitchen towel or paper towel. Remove any tough stems if required.
2. **Sauté Garlic:**
- Heat a drizzle of olive oil over medium heat in a big skillet or pan.
- Add the minced garlic and sauté for approximately 30 seconds to 1 minute until aromatic.
- Be cautious not to let the garlic brown.

3. **Add Spinach:** Add the cleaned and dried spinach leaves to the skillet. You may need to do this in batches since spinach cooks down rapidly.

4. **Sauté and mix:** Use tongs to mix the spinach in the garlic-infused oil gently. The heat will wilt the spinach down.

5. **Season:** Sprinkle a teaspoon of salt and pepper over the sautéed spinach. You may also add red pepper flakes for a hint of spiciness.

6. **Add Optional Ingredients:** Add a sprinkle of lemon zest or toasted pine nuts to the sautéed spinach for extra flavour and texture.

7. **Cook Until Wilted:** Continue sautéing the spinach for approximately 2-3 minutes or until it's wilted down and has decreased in volume.

8. **Serve:** Transfer the sautéed spinach to a serving dish. You may serve it as a side dish or as a basis for other meals.

Garlic sautéed spinach is a fast and nutrient-rich side that combines nicely with several main dishes. Spinach is an excellent source of vitamins and minerals, including vitamin K, essential for bone health. This recipe enhances joint health and general well-being with its basic but tasty ingredients.

# Greek Yogurt Cucumber Salad

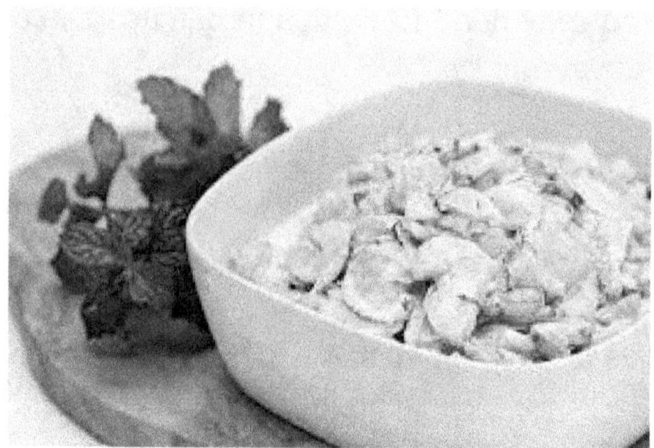

Ingredients:

- 2 cups Greek yogurt
- One cucumber peeled and diced
- ¼ red onion, coarsely chopped
- 1-2 cloves garlic, minced
- One tablespoon fresh dill, diced (or use dried dill)
- One tablespoon of fresh mint, chopped
- Juice of 1 lemon
- Salt & pepper, to taste
- Optional: crumbled feta cheese, chopped olives

Instructions:

1. **Prepare the Cucumber:** Peel it, if desired, and cut it into tiny pieces. You may also leave some skin on for extra texture and colour.

2. **Prepare the Dressing:** In a mixing dish, add Greek yoghurt, minced garlic, chopped dill, chopped mint, and lemon juice. Mix vigorously until the herbs and garlic are uniformly dispersed.

3. **Combine Ingredients:** Add the diced cucumber and finely chopped red onion to the yoghurt mixture. Mix the ingredients to coat the cucumber and onion with the yoghurt dressing.

4. **Season:** Season the cucumber salad with salt and pepper to taste. Adjust the seasoning according to your desire.

5. **Optional Additions:** Add crumbled feta cheese and chopped olives to the salad for added flavour if preferred.

6. **Chill and Serve:** Cover the bowl with plastic wrap or a cover and chill the cucumber salad for at least 30 minutes before serving. This enables the flavours to mingle and the salad to cool.

7. **Serve:** Before serving, give the salad a slight swirl. Serve the Greek Yogurt Cucumber Salad as a pleasant and creamy side dish.

This Greek Yogurt Cucumber Salad is tasty and has an excellent dose of protein and probiotics from the Greek yoghurt. Cucumbers are hydrating and contain vitamins that may assist in joint health and general well-being. The herbs and spices offer a burst of fresh flavour to the salad.


## Sautéed Mushrooms

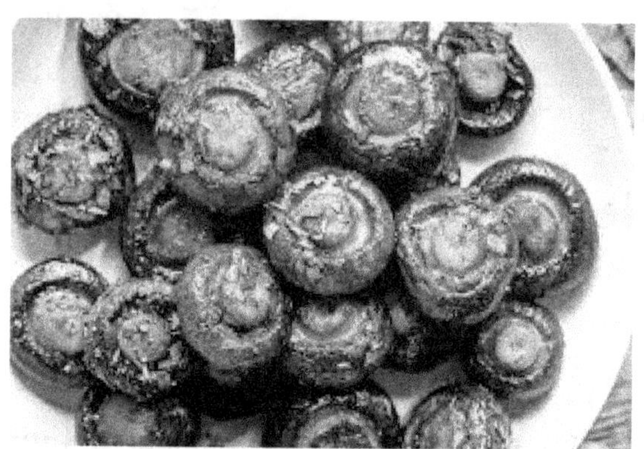

Ingredients:

- Fresh mushrooms (button, cremini, or your chosen variety), cleaned and sliced
- Butter or olive oil
- Garlic, minced
- Fresh thyme or rosemary leaves, chopped
- Salt & pepper, to taste
- Optional: splash of white wine or balsamic vinegar

Instructions:

1. **Prepare the Mushrooms:** Clean the mushrooms using a moist paper towel or a gentle brush to eliminate dirt. Slice the mushrooms to your chosen thickness.

2. **Heat the Pan:** Heat a tablespoon of butter or olive oil over medium-high heat in a skillet or pan.

3. **Sauté the Mushrooms:** Add the sliced mushrooms to the hot pan. Allow them to simmer without stirring for a few minutes. This helps them acquire a lovely sear.

4. **Add Flavor:** Once the mushrooms have begun to brown, add minced garlic and chopped fresh thyme or rosemary leaves. Stir everything together to disperse the flavours.

5. **Season:** Sprinkle salt and a dash of pepper over the mushrooms. Continue to sauté and stir occasionally.

6. **Optional Wine or Vinegar:** For extra depth of flavour, you may add a splash of white wine or balsamic vinegar to the mushrooms. Allow the liquid to reduce and coat the mushrooms.

7. **Cook Until soft:** Continue sautéing the mushrooms until they are soft and have a rich, golden-brown colour. This usually takes approximately 5-7 minutes.

8. **Serve:** Once the mushrooms are cooked to your taste, move them to a serving dish.

Sautéed mushrooms are a versatile side dish that adds depth and earthy flavour to your words. Mushrooms include minerals like selenium and antioxidants, which may help with joint health and general well-being. Customize the recipe using your preferred herbs and spices for a beautiful touch to your dish.


## Herbed Brown Rice

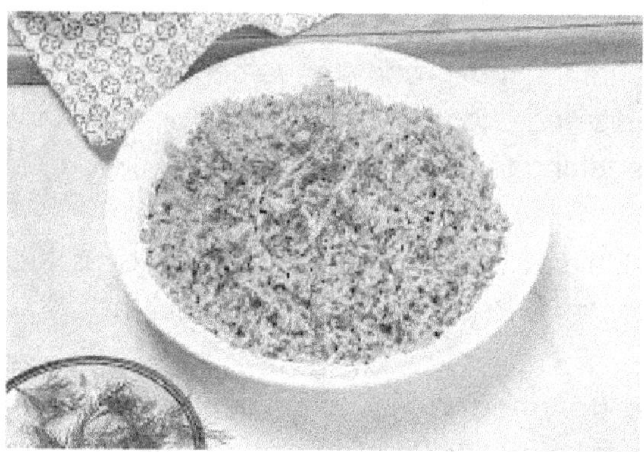

Ingredients:

- 1 cup brown rice
- 2 cups water or vegetable broth
- One tablespoon of olive oil or butter
- One teaspoon of dry herbs (such as thyme, rosemary, oregano, or a blend)
- Salt & pepper, to taste
- Fresh herbs (such as parsley or chives), chopped (for garnish)

Instructions:

1. **Rinse the Rice:** Rinse the brown rice under cold water until the water runs clear. This helps eliminate extra starch and prevents the rice from getting too sticky.

2. **Cook the Rice:**

- Mix the washed rice and water (or veggie broth) in a medium saucepan.
- Bring the mixture to a boil.
- Reduce the heat to low, cover the pot, and let the rice simmer for approximately 40-45 minutes or until the rice is cooked and the liquid is absorbed.

3. **Fluff the Rice:** Once the rice is done, remove the saucepan from the heat and let it rest, covered, for approximately 5 minutes. Then, use a fork to fluff the rice to separate the grains.

4. **Add Herbs and Seasoning:** Heat olive oil or butter over medium heat in a separate skillet or pan. Add the dry herbs and whisk for a minute until they become aromatic.

5. **Combine Rice and Herbs:** Add the cooked rice to the pan with the herbs and oil. Stir vigorously to spread the spices and oil among the rice properly.

6. **Season:** Season the herbed brown rice with salt and pepper to taste. Adjust the seasoning according to your desire.

7. **Garnish:** Before serving, add chopped fresh herbs (such as parsley or chives) over the herbed brown rice for an extra blast of flavour and colour.

Herbed brown rice is a nutritious and delicious side dish that compliments a range of main dishes. The herbs contribute to taste and possible anti-inflammatory properties that may promote joint health and general well-being. This recipe is a fantastic source of complex carbs and fibre, making it a healthful complement to your meals.


## Lemon Herb Roasted Asparagus

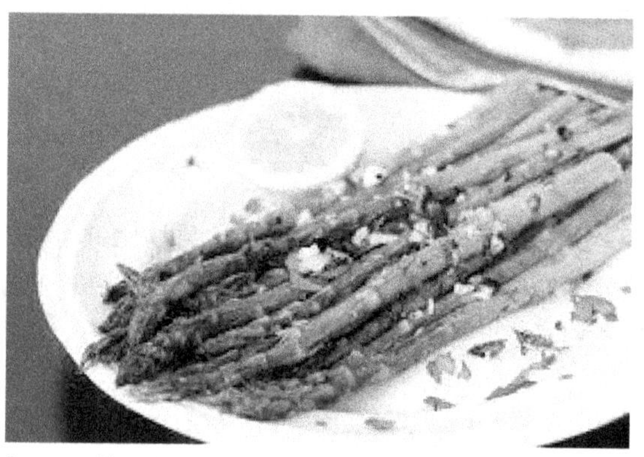

Ingredients:

- Fresh asparagus spears, trimmed Olive oil
- Zest of 1 lemon
- Juice of 1 lemon
- Fresh herbs (such as thyme, rosemary, or parsley), chopped
- Salt & pepper, to taste
- **Optional:** grated Parmesan cheese

1. **Preheat the Oven:** Preheat the oven to 400°F (200°C).

2. **Prepare the Asparagus:** Wash the spears and clip off the rough ends. You may snap off the woody ends or trim them where they naturally bend.

3. **Zest and Juice the Lemon:** Use a zester or a fine grater to zest the lemon. Then, squeeze the lemon and put aside the zest and JuiceJuiceJuice.

4. **Season and Coat:**
   - Place the trimmed asparagus stalks on a baking sheet.
   - Drizzle with olive oil, lemon juice, and lemon zest.
   - Toss the asparagus to coat them evenly with the oil and lemon.

5. **Add Herbs:** Sprinkle the chopped fresh herbs over the asparagus. The herbs will infuse the asparagus with flavour while they roast.

6. **Season:** Sprinkle salt and a dash of pepper over the asparagus to taste.

7. **Roast in the Oven:** Place the baking sheet in the oven and roast for approximately 12-15 minutes, or until the asparagus is tender but still a little crunchy. Cooking time may vary depending on the thickness of the asparagus.

8. **Optional Cheese:** If preferred, during the final few minutes of roasting, you may sprinkle grated Parmesan cheese over the asparagus for a delicious touch.

9. **Serve:** Transfer the roasted asparagus to a serving plate. Serve them heated as a tasty and nutrient-rich side dish.

Lemon Herb Roasted Asparagus is a tasty addition to meals and a source of vitamins and antioxidants. Asparagus includes elements that help improve joint health and general well-being. The lemon zest JuiceJuiceJuice and fresh herbs boost the meal with bright and fragrant tastes.

# CHAPTER EIGHT

## Indulgent but Anti-Inflammatory Desserts

## Dark Chocolate-Dipped Strawberries

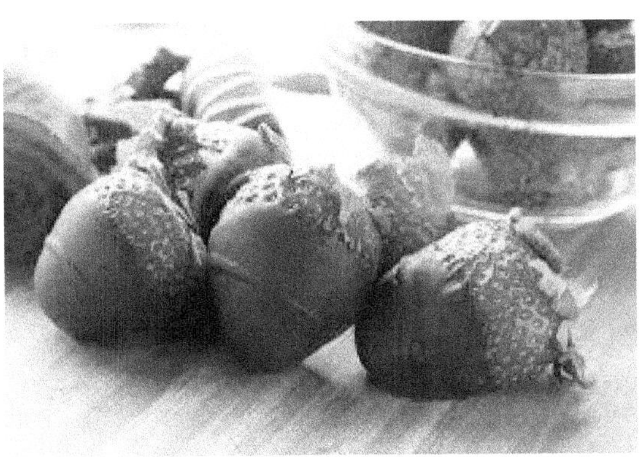

Ingredients:

- Fresh strawberries, cleaned and dried Dark chocolate (70% cocoa or higher), chopped
- Optional: coconut oil, chopped almonds, shredded coconut, sea salt

Instructions:

1. **Prepare the Strawberries:** Wash and thoroughly dry the strawberries. It's vital to dry them sufficiently to ensure the chocolate sticks correctly.

2. **Melt the Chocolate:** Place the chopped dark chocolate in a microwave-safe dish. Microwave in 20-30-second intervals, stirring after each interval, until the chocolate is thoroughly melted and smooth. You may alternatively melt the chocolate using a double boiler on the stovetop.

3. **Optional Coconut Oil:** If the melted chocolate appears a touch thick, you may add a tiny quantity of coconut oil to assist in producing a smoother dipping consistency. Stir well to mix.

4. **Dunk the Strawberries:** Hold a strawberry by the stem and dunk it into the melted chocolate, swirling to cover roughly two-thirds of the fruit. Lift the strawberry and let any extra chocolate fall off.

5. **Optional Toppings:** Before the chocolate hardens, roll the dipped strawberries in chopped almonds, shredded coconut, or a sprinkling of sea salt for extra taste and texture.

6. **Place on Parchment:** Place the chocolate-dipped strawberries on a parchment-lined tray or dish. Make sure they don't contact each other to avoid sticking.

7. **Chill:** Place the tray of dipped strawberries in the refrigerator for approximately 15-20 minutes or until the chocolate sets and hardens.

8. **Serve:** Move the dark chocolate-dipped strawberries to a serving plate once the chocolate is hardened. Enjoy as an indulgent and antioxidant-rich dessert.

Dark chocolate-dipped strawberries are a delicious delicacy that mixes the sweetness of ripe strawberries with dark chocolate's rich, somewhat bitter taste. Dark chocolate is recognized for its possible anti-inflammatory benefits owing to its high cocoa content. This meal enables you to fulfil your sweet desires while enjoying the potential health advantages of dark chocolate and strawberries.

## Chia Seed Pudding with Berries

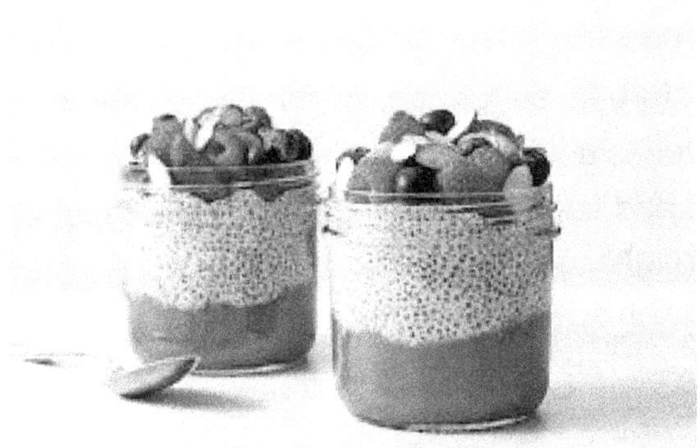

Ingredients:

- ¼ cup chia seeds
- 1 cup milk (dairy or plant-based)
- One tablespoon of honey or maple syrup (modify to taste)

- ½ teaspoon vanilla extract
- Fresh berries (strawberries, blueberries, raspberries)
- **Optional toppings:** chopped nuts, shredded coconut

Instructions:

1. **Mix Chia Seeds and Liquid:**
- Blend chia seeds and milk in a dish.
- Stir well to distribute the chia seeds properly.
- Make sure there are no clumps.

2. **Sweeten and Flavor:** Add honey or maple syrup and vanilla essence to the chia mixture. Stir to incorporate the sweetener and taste.

3. **Thicken:**
- Let the chia mixture settle for approximately 5 minutes.
- Stir again to avoid clumping.
- Cover the bowl and set it in the refrigerator for at least 2-3 hours or overnight.
- The chia seeds will absorb the liquid during this time and develop a pudding-like consistency.

4. **Toss and Serve:** Once the chia seed pudding has thickened, thoroughly toss it to break up any clumps. If the pudding is too thick, you may add a splash of milk to obtain your preferred consistency.

5. **Prepare Berries:** Wash and dry the fresh berries. If using strawberries, slice them.

6. **Assemble:** Spoon the chia seed pudding into serving bowls. Top with the fresh berries and any other toppings you choose, such as chopped almonds or shredded coconut.

7. **Serve:** Serve the Chia Seed Pudding with Berries as a healthful and pleasant dessert or breakfast alternative.

Chia seed pudding is tasty and rich in omega-3 fatty acids, fibre, and antioxidants. Including berries gives additional vitamins and antioxidants that help improve joint health and general well-being. Customize the recipe by picking your preferred milk and sweetener, and feel free to experiment with other fruit combinations and toppings.

## Baked Apples with Cinnamon

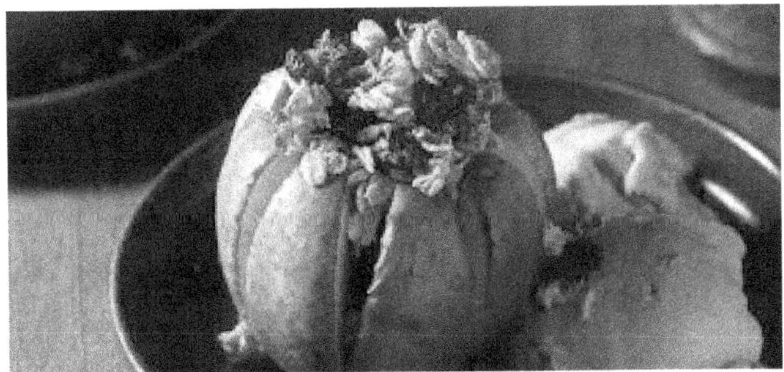

- Apples (firm and somewhat tart kinds such as Granny Smith or Honeycrisp)
- Ground cinnamon
- Honey or maple syrup (optional)
- Chopped nuts (such as walnuts or almonds)
- Raisins or dried cranberries (optional)
- Butter or coconut oil (optional)

## Instructions:

1. **Preheat the Oven:** Preheat the oven to 350°F (175°C).

2. **Prepare the Apples:** Wash the apples and then core them, either using an apple corer or gently removing the cores with a knife. Leave the bottom of the apples intact to accommodate the filling.

3. **Cinnamon Filling:** In a small dish, blend ground cinnamon with honey or maple syrup. The quantity of sweetness and cinnamon depends on your taste preferences.

4. **Fill the Apples:** Spoon the cinnamon mixture into the hollowed-out centres of the apples. Add a few raisins or dried cranberries to the filling for added sweetness and taste.

5. **Optional Butter or Oil:** For extra richness, sprinkle a little slice of butter or coconut oil on top of the filling in each apple.

6. **Bake:** Place the stuffed apples in a baking dish or sheet. Bake in the oven for approximately 25-30 minutes or until the apples are soft. You may verify their doneness by sticking a fork into the flesh - it should go in quickly.

7. **Serve:** Once roasted, remove the apples from the oven. Drizzle any syrup collected in the baking dish over the apples. Scatter chopped nuts over the top for crunch and extra flavour if desired.

8. **Enjoy:** Serve the Baked Apples with Cinnamon as a warm and pleasant dessert. You may eat them as they are or with a dollop of Greek yoghurt or a scoop of vanilla ice cream.

Baked apples with cinnamon are a delightful dessert choice that mixes the natural sweetness of apples with the warm flavour of cinnamon. Apples are a source of dietary fibre, antioxidants, and vitamins that aid in joint health and general well-being. This dessert is easy to create and may be adjusted to fit your taste preferences.

# Turmeric Golden Milk Popsicles

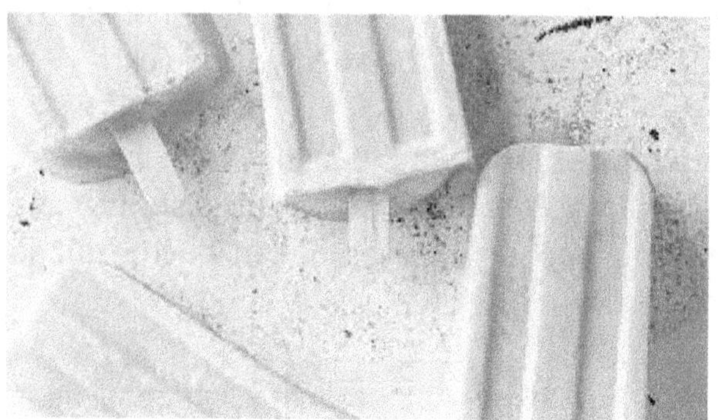



- 2 cups milk (dairy or plant-based)
- One teaspoon of ground turmeric
- ½ teaspoon ground cinnamon
- ¼ teaspoon ground ginger
- 1-2 tablespoons honey or maple syrup (modify to taste)
- Pinch of black pepper (to improve turmeric absorption)
- **Optional:** a sprinkle of ground cardamom or nutmeg

Instructions:

1. **Prepare the Golden Milk Mixture:**

- Heat the milk over medium heat in a saucepan until it's warm but not boiling.
- Add the ground turmeric, cinnamon, ginger, and a sprinkle of black pepper to the milk.
- Whisk the mixture until the spices are thoroughly mixed, and the milk becomes golden.

2. **Sweeten:** Add honey or maple syrup to the golden milk mixture, adjusting the quantity to your preferred degree of sweetness. Continue to whisk until the sweetener is entirely dissolved.

3. **Optional Spice:** If preferred, add a dash of ground cardamom or nutmeg for added taste.

4. **Cool and Pour:** Allow the golden milk mixture to cool before pouring it into popsicle moulds.

5. **Freeze:** Place the popsicle moulds in the freezer and let them freeze for 1-2 hours. After this period, place popsicle sticks into the moulds.

6. **Complete Freezing:** Allow the popsicles to freeze completely, generally for approximately 4-6 hours or overnight.

7. **Unmold and Serve:** Once the popsicles are frozen, take them from the moulds by gently running warm water over them to release the popsicles.

Enjoy the Turmeric Golden Milk Popsicles as a pleasant and anti-inflammatory treat. These popsicles mix the health of turmeric and spices with the cooling of frozen delights.

# Mixed Berry Parfait with Greek Yogurt

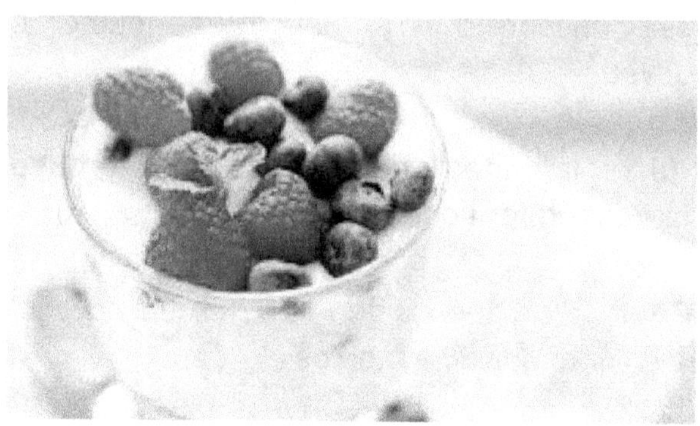



- Greek yoghurt (plain or vanilla-flavoured)
- Mixed berries (strawberries, blueberries, raspberries, blackberries)
- Honey or maple syrup (optional)
- Granola or chopped nuts (optional)
- Fresh mint leaves (for garnish, optional)

Instructions:

1. **Prepare the Berries:** Wash the berries and pat them dry with a paper towel. If using strawberries, remove the stems and slice them.

2. **Sweeten the Berries:** If desired, sprinkle honey or maple syrup over the berries to increase their sweetness. Toss lightly to coat the berries.

3. **Layer the Parfait:** Start by putting a layer of Greek yoghurt on the bottom of serving glasses or bowls.

4.  **Add Berries:** Add a layer of mixed berries to the yoghurt. You may alternate between various varieties of berries for a beautiful and tasty parfait.

5.  **Repeat Layers:** Continue stacking Greek yoghurt and mixed berries until you fill the glasses or bowls. You may build as many layers as you wish.

6.  **Top with Granola or Nuts:** For extra texture, sprinkle granola or chopped nuts on the berry layer.

7.  **Garnish:** Garnish the parfait with a few fresh mint leaves for a touch of freshness.

8.  **Serve:** Serve the Mixed Berry Parfait with Greek Yogurt as a healthful and enjoyable dessert or breakfast choice.

This parfait is rich in probiotics from Greek yoghurt and antioxidants from mixed berries. Berries are recognized for their possible anti-inflammatory properties, making this parfait a tasty and wholesome treat that improves joint health and general well-being. Customize the parfait with your preferred berries, yoghurt flavour, and toppings for a unique touch.

# Almond Flour Banana Bread

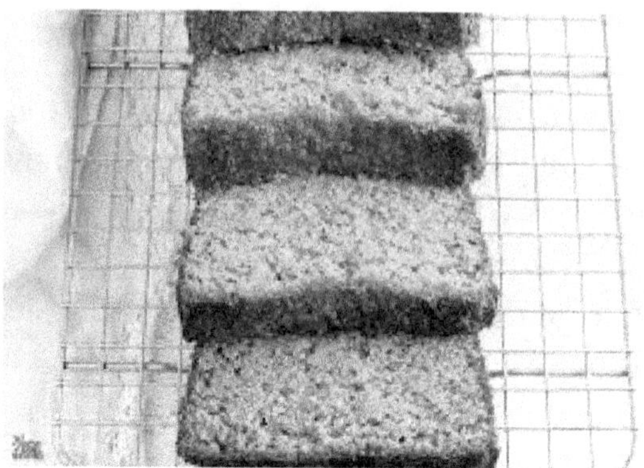

Ingredients:

- Three ripe bananas, mashed
- Three eggs
- ¼ cup melted coconut oil or butter
- One teaspoon of vanilla extract
- 2 cups almond flour
- One teaspoon of baking soda
- ½ teaspoon ground cinnamon
- Pinch of salt
- **Optional:** chopped nuts, chocolate chips, dried fruits

Instructions:

1. **Preheat the Oven:** Preheat the oven to 350°F (175°C). Grease a loaf pan or line it with parchment paper.

2. **Prepare Wet Ingredients:** In a mixing bowl, whisk together the mashed bananas, eggs, melted coconut oil or butter, and vanilla extract until thoroughly blended.

3. **Combine Dry Ingredients:** In a separate dish, whisk together the almond flour, baking soda, powdered cinnamon, and a touch of salt.

4. **Combine Wet and Dry:** Gradually add the dry component to the wet ingredients, stirring gently until the batter is thoroughly combined.

5. **Optional Add-Ins:** If preferred, stir chopped nuts, chocolate chips, or dried fruits into the batter for extra taste and texture.

6. **Transfer to Loaf Pan:** Pour the batter into the prepared loaf pan and distribute it evenly.

7. **Bake:** Place the loaf pan in the preheated oven and bake for approximately 45-55 minutes, or until a toothpick inserted into the middle of the bread comes out clean.

8. **Cool:** Once done, take the banana bread from the oven and allow it to cool in the pan for approximately 10-15 minutes. Then, transfer the bread to a wire rack to cool fully.

9. **Slice and Serve:** Once the banana bread is excellent, slice it into pieces and serve. Enjoy it as a delightful and nutrient-rich snack or dessert.

Almond flour banana bread is a gluten-free, lower-carb alternative to classic banana bread. Almond flour offers healthy fats, protein, and minerals, while bananas contribute natural sweetness and nutrition. This variation of banana bread is rich in taste and texture, and it may be a pleasant option for individuals trying to promote joint health and enjoy a nourishing treat.

## Avocado Chocolate Mousse

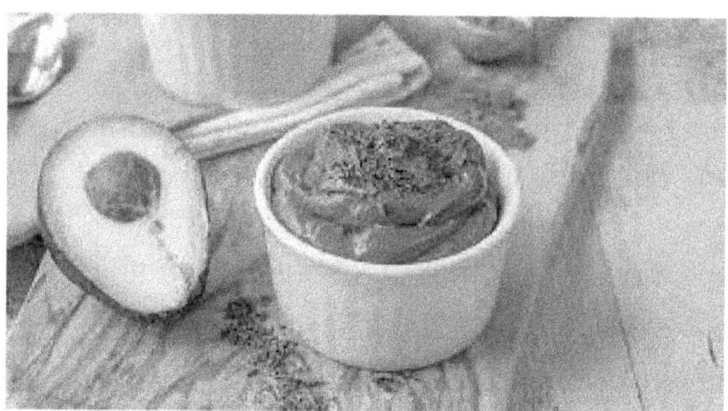

Ingredients:

- Two ripe avocados, peeled and pitted
- ¼ cup cocoa powder
- ¼ cup honey or maple syrup (adjust to taste)
- One teaspoon of vanilla extract
- Pinch of salt

- **Optional toppings:** whipped cream, shaved chocolate, berries

Instructions:

1. **Mix Avocado:** Mix the ripe avocados until smooth and creamy in a food processor or blender.

2. **Add Cocoa and Sweetener:** Add the cocoa powder, honey or maple syrup, vanilla essence, and a bit of salt to the pureed avocados.

3. **Blend Again:** Blend the mixture until all the elements are fully incorporated and the mousse is silky and smooth.

4. **Taste and Adjust:** Taste the chocolate mousse and adjust the sweetness or cocoa level according to your desire.

5. **Chill:** Transfer the chocolate mousse to serving dishes or glasses. Cover and refrigerate for at least 30 minutes to enable the flavours to mingle and the mousse to thicken.

6. **Serve:** Before serving, add extra toppings like a scoop of whipped cream, shaved chocolate, or fresh berries.

7. **Enjoy:** Serve the Avocado Chocolate Mousse as a rich and decadent dessert that contains the benefits of avocados' healthful fats and nutrients.

Avocado chocolate mousse is a healthier alternative to typical chocolate mousse since avocados give a creamy texture and beneficial fats. The natural sweetness from honey or maple syrup enhances the chocolate taste, making this dish both tasty and gratifying. Enjoy this indulgence in moderation as part of a healthy diet.


## Peach and Berry Crisp

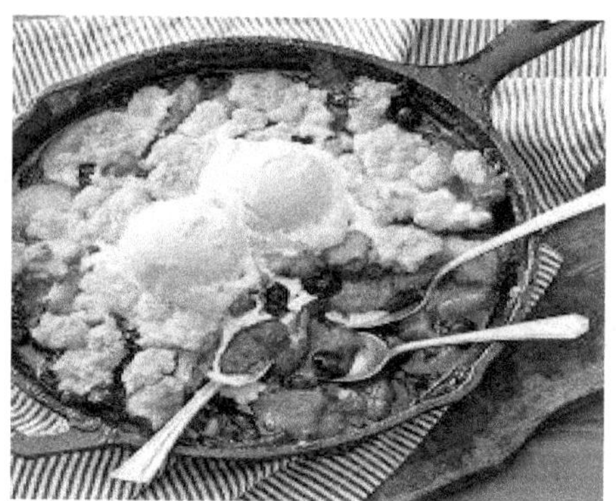

Ingredients:

For the Filling:

- 4 cups sliced fresh peaches (approximately 4-5 peaches)
- 1 cup mixed berries (blueberries, raspberries, blackberries)
- ¼ cup granulated sugar (adjust to taste)
- One tablespoon cornstarch
- One teaspoon of lemon juice
- ½ teaspoon vanilla extract

Pinch of salt For the Topping:

- 1 cup old-fashioned rolled oats
- ½ cup almond flour or all-purpose flour
- ¼ cup brown sugar
- ½ teaspoon ground cinnamon
- ¼ teaspoon salt
- ¼ cup cold unsalted butter, cubed
- **Optional:** chopped nuts (such as pecans or almonds)

Instructions:

1. **Preheat the Oven:** Preheat the oven to 350°F (175°C).

2. **Prepare the Filling:** In a mixing bowl, combine the sliced peaches, mixed berries, granulated sugar, cornstarch, lemon juice, vanilla essence, and a sprinkle of salt. Gently toss to coat the fruit with the sugar and cornstarch mixture.

3. **Transfer to Baking Dish:** Transfer the fruit mixture to a prepared baking dish or individual ramekins.

4. **Make the Topping:** In a separate dish, mix the rolled oats, almond flour or all-purpose flour, brown sugar, ground cinnamon, and salt. Add the cold cubed butter and use your fingers or a pastry cutter to knead the butter into the dry ingredients until the mixture resembles coarse crumbs. If using nuts, you may add them to the topping mixture.

5. **Top the Filling:** Sprinkle the oat and flour topping over the fruit mixture in the baking dish.

6. **Bake:** Place the baking dish in the oven for approximately 30-35 minutes, or until the fruit bubbles and the topping is golden brown.

7. **Cool Slightly:** Remove the crisp from the oven and let it cool slightly before serving.

8. **Serve:** Serve the Peach and Berry Crisp warm on its own or with a scoop of vanilla ice cream or a dollop of whipped cream.

Peach & Berry Crisp is a soothing dish that mixes the taste of juicy peaches and mixed berries with a crispy oat and flour topping. This dessert is rich in flavour, minerals, and antioxidants from the fruits, and it's excellent for savouring throughout the hot months.

# Coconut Rice Pudding

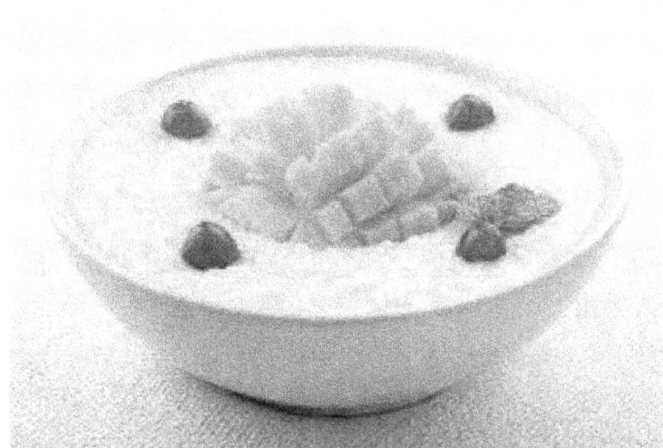

Ingredients:

- 1 cup Arborio rice (or other short-grain rice)
- 2 cups water
- One can (13.5 oz) coconut milk (full-fat)
- ¼ cup granulated sugar (adjust to taste)
- ½ teaspoon vanilla extract
- Pinch of salt
- Optional: toasted coconut flakes, chopped almonds, dried fruit, ground cinnamon

Instructions:

1. **Rinse the Rice:** Rinse the Arborio rice under cold water until the water runs clear. This helps eliminate extra starch and prevents the rice pudding from getting too sticky.

2. **Cook the Rice:** In a medium saucepan, mix the rinsed rice and water. Bring the mixture to a boil, then decrease

the heat to low, cover the pot, and let the rice simmer for approximately 15 minutes, or until the rice is essentially cooked and the water is absorbed.

3. **Add Coconut Milk:** Add coconut milk to the cooked rice saucepan. Stir well to mix.

4. **Sweeten and Flavor:** Add granulated sugar, vanilla essence, and salt to the rice and coconut milk combination. Stir to dissolve the sugar and integrate the seasonings.

5. **Continue Cooking:** Simmer the rice pudding over low heat, stirring often, until the rice is thoroughly cooked and the mixture has thickened. This will take roughly 20-25 minutes.

6. **Optional Add-Ins:** If preferred, add toasted coconut flakes, chopped nuts, dried fruit, or a sprinkling of ground cinnamon to the rice pudding for extra texture and taste.

7. **Cool and Serve:** Once the rice pudding has achieved your preferred consistency, remove it from the pan and cool slightly. Serve it warm, or chill it and enjoy it cold.

8. **Serve:** Serve the Coconut Rice Pudding as a creamy and decadent dessert or brunch choice.

Coconut rice pudding is a soothing and creamy dish that mixes the richness of coconut milk with the comforting taste of rice.

Coconut milk delivers healthful fats and a tropical flavour, while rice lends a pleasing texture. Customize the recipe with your favourite add-ins and toppings to make a dessert that meets your taste preferences.

## Walnut Date Bites

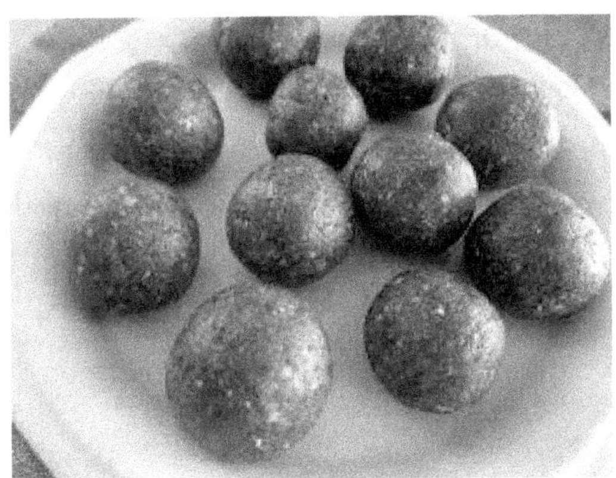

Ingredients:

- 1 cup pitted dates
- 1 cup walnuts
- ¼ teaspoon ground cinnamon
- Pinch of salt
- **Optional:** cocoa powder, shredded coconut, vanilla extract

Instructions:

1. **Process Dates:** In a food processor, add pitted dates, walnuts, ground cinnamon, and a touch of salt.

2. **Blend:** Process the ingredients until they are thoroughly blended, and the mixture begins to come together. It should have a sticky consistency.

3. **Optional Add-Ins:** Depending on your desire, add a teaspoon of cocoa powder for chocolate flavour or a dash of vanilla essence for added scent.

4. **Form Bites:** Scoop tiny parts of the mixture and roll them into bite-sized balls using your hands. Press and shape the mixture firmly to keep its form.

5. **Coat or Garnish:** For extra flavour and texture, you may roll the walnut date nibbles in shredded coconut, chocolate powder, or broken nuts.

6. **Chill:** Place the walnut date bits on a dish or tray and fridge them for approximately 30 minutes to firm up.

7. **Store:** Transfer the bites to an airtight container once they are cold. Store them in the refrigerator for freshness.

8. **Enjoy:** Enjoy the Walnut Date Bites as a fast and naturally sweet snack that delivers a blend of healthy fats and natural sugars.

Walnut date bites are a nutrient-rich snack that blends dates' natural sweetness with walnuts' crunchiness. Dates supply natural sugars for energy, while walnuts add healthful fats and protein. These bites may be a delightful and practical alternative to keep on hand when you need a fast and healthy snack.

# CHAPTER NINE

## Cooking Techniques for Preserving Nutrients

## Steaming, Roasting, and Grilling Tips

Steaming:

1. **Choose the Right Equipment:** Use a steamer basket, bamboo steamer, or a microwave-safe dish with a cover to steam your meal.

2. **Add Flavors:** Enhance the taste of your steamed foods by adding herbs, spices, citrus zest, or even a dash of broth to the water.

3. **Control the Steam:** Make sure the water simmer and does not boil furiously. Too much heat may cause overcooking.

4. **Timing:** Different meals need different steaming periods. Harder veggies could take longer than delicate fish or shellfish. Keep an eye on the cooking process.

5. **Check Doneness:** Test the doneness of your meal by inserting a fork or knife. It should glide in effortlessly with minimum resistance.

1. **Preheat the Oven:** Ensure your oven is preheated to the proper temperature before roasting.

2. **Use the Right Pan:** Choose a baking sheet or roasting pan with enough room to enable the food to cook evenly.

3. **Spread Evenly:** Spread the food in a single layer to achieve even cooking and browning.

4. **Oil and Seasoning:** Toss the food with oil and your choice of spices to improve taste and encourage browning.

5. **Monitor and Rotate:** Keep an eye on the roasting process and rotate the pan if required to avoid uneven browning.

6. **Check Internal Temperature:** For meats, use a meat thermometer to confirm they're cooked to the proper internal temperature.

Grilling:

1. **Preheat the Grill:** Preheat your grill to a suitable temperature before cooking.

2. **Clean and Oil the Grates:** Clean the grates and brush them with oil to avoid sticking.

3. **Direct and Indirect Heat:** Understand the difference between direct heat (over the flames) and indirect heat (to the side of the fire). Use these zones to alter the cooking speed.

4. **Marinate or Season:** Marinating meats or veggies may add flavour and help tenderize. Seasoning with salt and pepper before grilling is vital.

5. **Use Skewers or Grill Baskets:** Skewers are fantastic for kebabs, while grill baskets prevent smaller foods from dropping through the grates.

6. **Flare-ups:** Be prepared for flare-ups from drippings by having a spray bottle of water available to suppress fires.

7. **Rest Meat:** Allow cooked meats to rest before slicing.

8. This helps preserve liquids and provides uniform dispersion of tastes.

Remember that each cooking process has particular advantages and tastes, so experiment to discover what works best for various items. Practice and experience will help you perfect your steaming, roasting, and grilling abilities to make tasty and healthful meals.

# Healthy Oil Alternatives

1. **Olive Oil:** Extra virgin olive oil is high in monounsaturated fats and antioxidants. It's perfect for salad dressings, sautéing, and mild cooking.

2. **Coconut Oil:** Unrefined coconut oil includes medium-chain triglycerides (MCTs) and has a faint coconut taste. It's excellent for baking, sautéing, and low-heat cooking.

3. **Avocado Oil:** Avocado oil has a high smoke point and is rich in monounsaturated fats and vitamin E. It's great for high-heat cooking, grilling, and roasting.

4. **Grapeseed Oil:** Grapeseed oil has a high smoke point and a moderate taste. It's ideal for sautéing, stir-frying, and baking.

5. **Sesame Oil:** Toasted sesame oil lends a particular taste to Asian foods. Use it sparingly and mainly as a finishing oil for flavour.

6. **Flaxseed Oil:** Flaxseed oil is abundant in omega-3 fatty acids. However, it's best used as a drizzle over meals after cooking since it's heat-sensitive.

7. **Walnut Oil:** Walnut oil offers a nutty taste and is a high source of omega-3 fatty acids. Use it in salad dressings or as a finishing oil.

8.  **Canola Oil:** Canola oil has a high smoke point and is low in saturated fat. It's ideal for frying, baking, and regular cooking.

9.  **Sunflower Oil:** Sunflower oil has a neutral taste and a high smoke point. It's adaptable for cooking, baking, and frying.

10. **Peanut Oil:** Peanut oil has a high smoke point and is often used in Asian cuisines for stir-frying and deep-frying.

11. **Hemp Oil:** Hemp oil is rich in omega-3 and omega-6 fatty acids. Like flaxseed oil, it's best used as a finishing oil.

12. **Rice Bran Oil:** Rice bran oil has a high smoke point and a moderate taste. It's ideal for numerous culinary techniques, including frying and sautéing.

When picking a cooking oil, consider the smoke point, taste, and nutritional profile that best meets your culinary demands. Using various oils to benefit from diverse nutrients and flavours is also a good idea. Keep in mind that moderation is crucial since all oils are calorie-dense.

# CHAPTER TEN

## Long-Term Strategies for Rheumatoid Arthritis Management

## Lifestyle Changes for Continued Relief

1. **Maintain a Healthy Diet:** Continue following an anti-inflammatory diet rich in fruits, vegetables, whole grains, lean meats, and healthy fats. Minimize processed meals, sugary snacks, and foods rich in saturated fats.

2. **Frequent Exercise:** Use low-impact workouts, such as swimming, walking, and mild yoga. Exercise helps preserve joint flexibility, minimize stiffness, and enhance overall strength.

3. **Weight Management:** Maintain a healthy weight to prevent unnecessary joint stress. Losing weight, if required, may ease joint discomfort and improve mobility.

4. **Stay Hydrated:** Drink lots of water to keep your body and joints hydrated. Proper hydration helps joint lubrication and general well-being.

5. **Mindful Stress Management:** Practice stress-reduction strategies such as meditation, deep breathing,

awareness, or gentle stretching. Chronic stress may increase inflammation and discomfort.

6. **Adequate Sleep:** Prioritize quality sleep to help the body's healing and repair processes. Aim for 7-9 hours of sound sleep each night.

7. **Joint Protection:** Be attentive to your joint motions and employ ergonomic tools, good body mechanics, and mutual protection measures to decrease strain.

8. **Regular Medical checks:** Continue to visit your healthcare practitioner periodically for reviews and modifications to your treatment plan as required.

9. **Medication Management:** Adhere to your prescription drugs and work closely with your healthcare practitioner to check their efficacy and possible adverse effects.

10. **Social Support:** Maintain ties with friends, family, and support groups. Emotional well-being may play a key role in treating chronic diseases.

11. **Adaptive Tools:** Use adaptive tools or equipment to make everyday chores easier on your joints, such as jar openers, ergonomic utensils, and assistive devices.

12. **Stay Informed:** Keep up with the newest advancements in rheumatoid arthritis management, including new medicines, lifestyle measures, and self-care practices.

Remember that every individual's experience with rheumatoid arthritis might be unique, so it's crucial to adjust these lifestyle modifications to your requirements and preferences. Consistency in keeping these modifications may lead to long-term alleviation and an enhanced quality of life. Discuss with your healthcare professional before substantially changing your lifestyle or treatment plan.

## Creating Balanced Meal Plans

Creating balanced meal plans requires consuming various nutrients from various food categories to enhance general health and well-being. Here's a guide to help you develop flat meal plans:

1. Include a Variety of Food Groups:
   - ✓ **Proteins:** Include lean proteins such as chicken, fish, lean meats, eggs, tofu, beans, and lentils.
   - ✓ **Carbohydrates:** Opt for whole grains such as brown rice, quinoa, whole wheat pasta, and whole grain bread.
   - ✓ **Healthy Fats:** Choose sources like avocados, nuts, seeds, olive oil, and fatty seafood.
   - ✓ **Veggies:** Incorporate a variety of colourful veggies for vitamins, minerals, and fibre.
   - ✓ **Fruits:** Include a variety of fresh, frozen, or dried fruits for natural sweetness and micronutrients.
   - ✓ **Dairy or Dairy Alternatives:** Choose low-fat or plant-based calcium and vitamin D choices.

## 2. Portion Control:

- ✓ Aim for balanced servings that give necessary nutrition without overdoing.
- ✓ **Use your hand as a guide:** Protein (palm-sized piece), Carbohydrates (fist-sized part), Healthy Fats (thumb-sized portion), and Vegetables (2 fists).

## 3. Prioritize Nutrient Density:

- ✓ Choose nutrient-dense meals that give a lot of vitamins, minerals, and antioxidants per calorie.
- ✓ Include a variety of coloured fruits and vegetables to acquire a range of nutrients.

## 4. Fiber-Rich Foods:

Include fibre-rich foods, including whole grains, vegetables, fruits, legumes, and nuts.
Fiber improves digestion, increases satiety, and supports heart health.

## 5. Hydration:

- Drink lots of water throughout the day to keep hydrated.
- Herbal teas, infused water, and low-sugar drinks also aid in hydration.

## 6. Balanced Meals:

- Aim for balanced meals that contain protein, complex carbs, healthy fats, and lots of veggies.
- A balanced lunch helps normalize blood sugar levels and delivers prolonged energy.

### 7. Plan:

- ✓ Plan meals to ensure you have balanced selections accessible.
- ✓ Batch cooking and meal preparation may save time and make healthy choices more accessible.

### 8. Snack Wisely:

- ✓ Choose nutrient-dense snacks like Greek yoghurt, vegetables with hummus, a handful of almonds, or a piece of fruit.
- ✓ Avoid excessive munching on empty-calorie meals.

### 9. Mindful Eating:

- ✓ Eat consciously, paying attention to hunger and fullness signs.
- ✓ Avoid distractions when eating to improve digestion and enjoyment.

### 10. Moderation and Variety:

- ✓ Practice moderation with delights and pleasures.
- ✓ Include a variety of foods to minimize vitamin deficits and make meals enjoyable.

Everyone's dietary requirements are unique, so consider visiting a certified dietitian or healthcare expert for tailored counsel. Creating balanced meal planning may assist in supporting your general health, energy levels, and particular health objectives.